MORPHOLOGY

Published collaboratively by Violet Pigeone Productions
and Tropos School of Classical Midwifery and Homeopathy

ISBN: 978-0-578-27868-1

First printing: 2023

MORPHOLOGY

Embodiment
and its significance
for Midwifery,
Homeopathy
and the
Manifestation of Presence

Molly Caliger

Dedication and thanks

This book has undergone numerous revisions as I gathered more obser-vations and experience through the years. I wish to express deep grat-itude to friends and acquaintances without whom this book would not have been written: my family, on all sides of the oceans and the Great Divide; Dr. Anatoly Nikolaev, my dear friend and obstetric mentor; the late Misha Norland and Edward Whitmont, who, among others, gave me a solid homeopathic foundation; all past and present pregnant and birthing women whom I have been honored to help; my homeopathy patients; all of my students and colleagues of Tropos School who have kept my head above water for many years; Patsy Rodenburg, who has gifted me with a new context for my work; and of course above all I thank our merciful and loving God.

Contents

Introduction

This book came into being as a product of many years' study and experience working with people and their bodies in various contexts. The material contained herein is a compilation of knowledge I have collected and personal experience I have gained while working first as a midwife and later as a homeopath. Still later I was given the opportunity to expand my insights while working with people interested in learning how to be *present*, in order to find and use their *voices*: women, men, parents, children, elderly, disabled, doctors and healthcare specialists, clergy, executives, actors, performers, and my own patients and students—with all kinds of ailments. In this book I offer a unique and holistic approach to understanding people more deeply by looking at their morphology: their individual shape and form. It is a system that can be applied in any of the healing arts (especially midwifery and homeopathy) as well as in any field whose aim is to help people reach their maximum in becoming who they are.

Experience has taught me that the pelvis is relevant not only for midwifery and childbirth, but also as the key to the entire morphological mosaic. Its significance as the seat of sexuality, creation, and new life is a given, but the detail it can reveal about an individual is wondrous. It is the key to understanding a person's tendencies, latent or expressed, and therefore is irreplaceable for making prognoses and understanding constitution and miasms[1], personality and psychology, potential course

---

1   miasm: in homeopathy, a group of hereditary tendencies, latent or potential symptoms and illnesses within a spectrum of potential illnesses, with which one is born.

of labor and childbirth, ease or difficulty in being present, ability to discover and use the natural voice to full capacity, and facility with forming meaningful relationships.

The body has been given bad press over the years as being either superfluous to the soul (in relation to which it is often considered inferior), or irrelevant to the human being in question. This assumption couldn't be farther from the truth. In this book I hope to demonstrate and prove the significance of the body as the external manifestation of a person's being and essence. Moreover, I hope to convince you of the relevance of specific body patterns for the understanding of the person as a whole.

This information can be applied by anyone, but is especially valuable for those in the healing arts. For midwives, obstetricians, and other childbirth professionals interested in facilitating normal physiological birth, this knowledge is indispensable. For holistic and complementary practitioners such as homeopaths, osteopaths, chiropractors, and massage therapists, as well as psychologists, physical therapists, neurologists, and every other specialty, this knowledge will undoubtedly open up a whole new way of understanding the person. Such an understanding should assist in arriving at preventive and curative therapies, exercises, and recommendations appropriate to each individual person. Those involved in performing arts, whether as performers or teachers, can greatly benefit from this knowledge as it holds the key to a wider understanding of the reasons behind various blockages and difficulties. For actors and directors, it can be a wellspring of inspiration for deeper understanding of roles and the actors who play them. Such professionals can use this knowledge to better understand the advantages and limitations of each morphological type in relation to body carriage, bodily ability to be present, use of breath and breath capacity, and the range, pitch, and even quality of the voice.

The book includes detailed descriptions of the morphological types, and how to identify each. There is discussion about the correspondence between morphology, labor and birth, psychological and character tendencies, predispositions, homeopathic constitutions and miasms, body posture and carriage, ability to speak and be heard and to hear others. Finally, I provide recommendations specific to each morphological type for working with the specific obstacles in each area.

I formulated this morphological system beginning with my work in Russian maternity hospitals from 1992 to 2005. During those years I directed an internship program for American midwifery students in six maternity hospitals of St. Petersburg, where over the course of 13 years approximately 100 students completed the three-month internship. The organization was founded at the tail end of the first Cold War and it was called The Russian Birth Project. Originally I created it with the desire to facilitate communication and friendship between Americans and Russians on the "field" of childbirth. Such a field has no place for wars, be they cold or unspoken; a birthing woman is in her most intimate place, where full presence of all involved is required. During those years in the maternity hospitals, I learned what turned out to be the last remnants of *classical midwifery*. I had many teachers, but the one who taught me more than anyone else is my close friend Dr. Anatoly Nikolaev. Some of the pearls of knowledge described herein came from Anatoly, others from very old midwifery texts or from elderly Russian midwives, while another part comes from Western obstetrics of the 19th and early 20th centuries. Experience with birthing women and with homeopathic patients provided valuable insights into the connection between morphology and constitution. Finally, I began integrating the connections between morphology and one's presence while studying with one of the world's leading voice teachers, Patsy Rodenburg, without whose inspiration I would not have expanded this book.

There are many specific terms used in the book, most of which derive from either classical midwifery or homeopathy. Each term is explained along the way. I am always interested in receiving feedback from readers after they begin to apply this work. Every contribution to the data pool serves to further our shared understanding and experience.

CHAPTER ONE.

Morphology and its significance

What? Know ye not that your body is the
Temple of the Holy Spirit which is in you, which ye have of God,
And ye are not your own?

Corinthians 6:19

Morphology (from the Greek μορφή "form" and λογία "science") in the widest sense of the term refers to the science of form and structure. Human morphology has been up until now almost exclusively limited to the study of discrete parts. In midwifery, for example, pelvimetry concerns itself with the study of the female pelvis and the bony and muscular structures of the pelvic floor. In classical homeopathy, attention is paid to body type and appearance, but only in the most general way. Western medicine acknowledges body type in relation to predisposition to certain diseases, but only in passing. The sense that this book ascribes to morphology is a new approach in health and healing. It posits that morphology is more than all that: it is the study of the human body not only in relation to itself, but as reflection of the whole person.

Morphology, as revealed in the totality of the body, is the visible, tangible part of the person. It represents the expression of the person's essence incarnated. It is the idea of the person manifested as *word*—as explicate form of implicate information crystallized in space and time. What we observe, then, in one's morphology, reveals the truest nature of a person. One can alter one's external appearance with cosmetics and even surgery, but it is more difficult to change the distance between one's eyes, the shape of the jaw, the level of the hairline, the degree of hairiness, the tendency toward well-defined muscles or a flaccid physique, the thickness of the bones. Morphology provides the tangible reflection of the divine image in its unique expression in the individual.

When we examine a person's rhombus of Michaelis (to be discussed in detail in later chapters), study the shape of the legs and the proportions of the body parts, note where the most weight is accumulated, observe the wrists to uncover the overall bone mass, and make several other casual observations in the course of five minutes—we are able to make certain hypotheses about the person: about past, present, and potentially future health issues and predispositions to disease; about likes and dislikes, passions and aversions; about character traits and values; about the person's degree of presence with self and others; about difficulties in self-expression; about intimacy and sexuality; and of course, in the case of a woman—about the potential course of her pregnancy, labor, and birth. This is possible owing to the phenomenon of hierarchical reflexion: something on one level holds within itself the characteristics of something else on another level. The macrocosm is contained within the microcosm and vice versa. The universe is reflected in an atom. As Hermes Trismegistus wrote: "As above, so below, as within, so without, as the universe, so the soul." What is proposed here is much more than simple reflexology—insofar as the body contains a certain hierarchy within itself just as does the whole of creation. This can only be true, since a person is more than the sum of the parts. A person is a totality. Yet even that term falls short of the explanation. The totality of a person— or indeed any totality—is like a hologram; the whole is enfolded in the details. Morphologically, there are certain key parts that are more significant than others for understanding the whole. This simplifies our work. Rather than examine a person under a microscope endlessly, carefully noting every detail, of which there are always more to uncover—we look at the keys, what I term the "skeleton" of the case. This is genuine holistic practice. Holistic thinking is not just about acknowledging the significance of the body, mind, and spirit and then treating each category separately. It is about gaining a feeling for the parts of a system and uncovering their place in the whole, and, even more significantly, gaining a relatively accurate comprehension of the whole from what the parts tell us. People can have mystical personal experiences of God in visions, and they can equally also feel God's presence in the splendor of nature, the overcoming of a struggle, in the synchronicity of significant events, or in the chance meeting of a "perfect" stranger. A person, as a unified whole, as a totality which is more than the sum of its parts, is not a machine. A person can only develop, and grow, and heal, and create, and become, as a whole. This applies to every person in every context.

Certain parts and their qualities are more representative than others for identifying the totality. The whole of creation exists in a hierarchy and the body does, as well. Hierarchical organization can be observed on every level: within one single person, as well as between the classes of beings on the earth, from mineral to micro-organism to plant to fish to insect to birds to animals to humans, and then upward into the higher spheres of the celestial hierarchy of the nine orders of angels[2] and finally reaching God. Reflection—that is, recognizing a trait or a symptom of the whole from one of the parts—is only possible because of the similarity between the levels of the hierarchy of creation[3]. But it remains a task to discover that reflection and identify those connections, which is only accomplished through intense observation and attention. The understanding of the whole in the parts and the parts as individual expressions of the whole far precedes the modern era. The ancient Christian Church based its original teachings on the fundamental truth taken from Genesis 1:27: *So God created man in his own image, in the image of God created he him; male and female created he them.* Our modern world is thankfully making attempts to recover what was forgotten since Descartes's vision of a clockwork universe and the mass migration of consciousness into the

---

2   Dionysios the Areopagite. "The Celestial Hierarchy." Available at: http://www. esoteric.msu.edu/VolumeII/CelestialHierarchy.html
3   Helmig, Christoph and Carlos Steel, "Proclus", *The Stanford Encyclopedia of Philosophy* (Fall 2021 Edition), Edward N. Zalta (ed.). Available at: https://plato. stanford.edu/archives/fall2021/entries/proclus/>.

discrete and the finite for its own sake. It requires that we learn to be *present* with ourselves, each other, and all of creation, so that our capacity for observation might be better honed. This is a tall order in the 21st century when virtual communication and distanced interaction predominate.

Working with fellow human beings on our earthly pilgrimage and putting ourselves in positions of healer, midwife, teacher, or coach, we must begin with a question: what do I want for this person whom I am desiring to help? The answer is not necessarily a given. It certainly concerns ethics; ethics always entails the whole. A relationship is about more than the mere interaction between two persons; a true relationship is continually giving birth to a third element, the "child," resulting as the product of presence and love. This awareness entails connection between the levels of creation. We don't need to necessarily see the divine spark at the core of every being, but we need to know that it's there. Such a faith keeps us moving toward a positive result and our faith is sensed by those with whom we work. This is entailed in presence. As one author described the thought of Plato: "Humans who understand the workings of the cosmos become not just spectators of, but participants in, divine reason and can ascend to the heavenly realm and attain again the divine vision. In order to do this, souls must live ethical lives. Ethics is inextricably connected with teleology and the return of the soul to its home."[4] There can be no holistic (and therefore no truly healing) practice of any sort without an acknowledgment that all beings are connected in a hierarchical fashion—just as the body has its hierarchy of function and form—and that all human beings make up the major elements of our earthly organism, or what Plato termed the world-soul, the *animus mundi*. These truths were self-evident for the great majority of human history.

---

4   Gabriela Roxana Carone, *Plato's Cosmology and its Ethical Dimensions* (New York: Cambridge University Press, 2005).

Undertaking our task and how it is to be accomplished demands of us a solid philosophical-theoretical position regarding the human person. We must know, with a high level of certainty, what we are doing, what our intention is, and what may be the probable reactions, before we take upon ourselves the responsibility of assisting others in their processes.

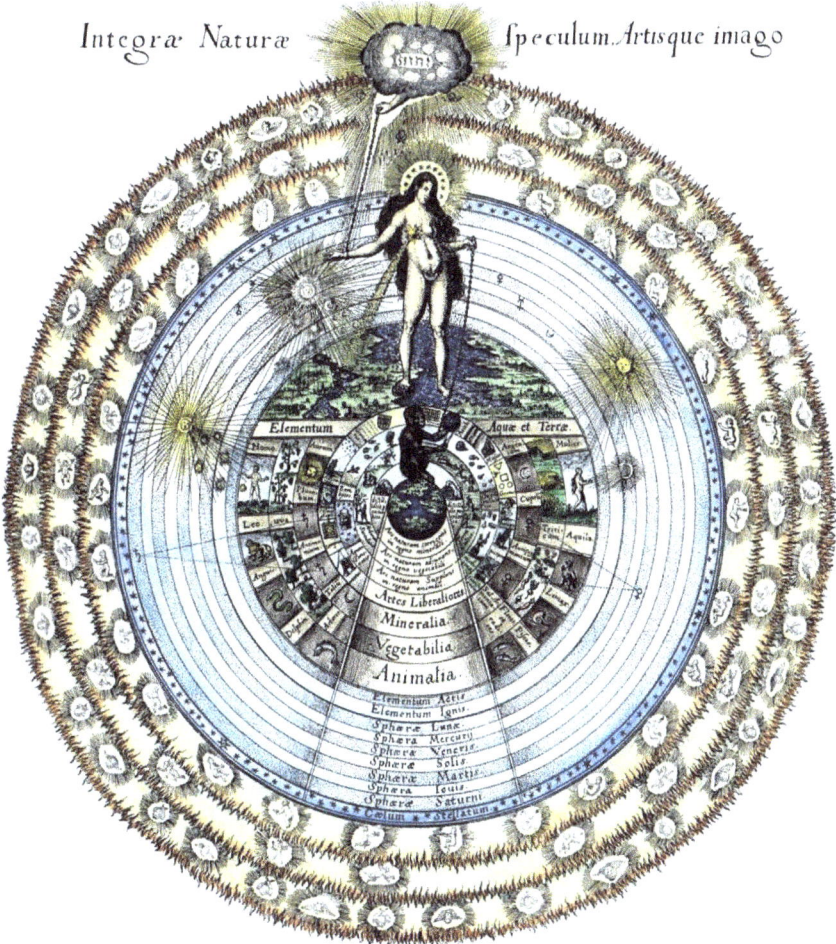

16th century illustration of the correspondences between all parts of the created cosmos, with the anima mundi depicted as a woman, from the *Utriusque cosmi maioris scilicet et minoris metaphysica, physica atque technica historia* by Robert Fludd.

The Soul

The trinitarian nature of the person has been described since ancient times as divided into body, spirit, and soul. Various terms for the threesome are used and the definitions are confusing, especially in regard to the "soul." The soul is also called the *nous* (from the Greek νοῦς[5] = mind), although in English that term does not quite convey the meaning originally attributed to this aspect of the person both by the ancient Greeks and by Eastern Orthodox Christianity. Contemporary holistic practitioners use the term "body-mind," which is a bi-level rather than a trinitarian interpretation. For homeopaths, the soul is the level of thought processes, the mental sphere: one's overall cognition or relationship to and understanding of the world. It includes thoughts, interpretations, opinions, values, beliefs, preferences, aversions, assessment. The mental and emotional spheres are usually referred to collectively as the psyche. The ancient Church[6] fathers and mothers called the *nous* the "eye of the heart or soul" or the "mind of the heart". It is the cognitive faculty, and more—the soul is that which holds the person together in one whole.

The soul is regarded by many traditions as the eternal part of the human being which can never be completely destroyed and continues its existence even after one's earthly death. In health and illness too, the soul is the deepest level of the person's being. When the soul is afflicted, a person questions existence itself, or is incapable of rational thought, and the farther away the soul strays, the more vulnerable one is to physical death (dementia, Alzheimer's, alcoholism, drug abuse, psychosis, etc.). Many pre-Christian ancient religious systems had similar beliefs about the soul. The shamans of Siberia believe that illness happens when the soul wanders far from the body, and the shaman's job is to retrieve it.

---

5   Archimandrite Georgios Abbot of the Holy Monastery of St. Gregorios On Mount Athos, "The Neptic and Hesychastic Character of Orthodox Athonite Monasticism." Available at: www.greekorthodoxchurch.org/neptic_monasticism.html

6   The "ancient Church" refers to the original church of the early Christians, which developed in the first centuries after Jesus Christ's resurrection and had its seat in the Byzantine empire until the schism of 1054 which divided the Church into western and eastern branches (i.e., Roman Catholicism and Eastern Orthodox).

The ancient Christian Church regards the soul as having been created by God, for all eternity.

The Judeo-Christian tradition teaches that each person—made of soul, spirit, and body—is created in God's image. According to the ancient Church fathers and mothers, the divine image of each person was tainted after the fall into sin. All people sin, and alter the divine image within themselves, and have the ultimate life purpose of restoring their godly image as closely as possible while they live on the earth. The ancient Church calls this the process of *theosis*. There is a similar concept in contemporary psychotherapy called actualization. Theosis brings one closer to the divine and true self. This means that the God-man Jesus Christ, as the most perfect *simillimum* of the human person, is also the universal homeopathic remedy for all of humankind. The Eucharist—taking the body and blood of Christ—is thus the perfect homeopathic medicine for the human soul, intensifying as does any homeopathic remedy those symptoms which are similar to the remedy (in this case the divine aspects of ourselves), working in us to encourage and enable our theosis.

The Spirit

The spirit is derived from the original "breath of God" breathed into the human person from the moment of creation. It is the Holy Spirit in us. This spirit in us reflects the degree and quality of *inspiration* we experience. Inspiration is literally the "breathing in" of divine grace: the gifts surrounding us in all of creation. Our inspiration provides motivation for life. It is revealed and reflected in our feeling states. Feelings, too, exist in a hierarchy: from the depth of despair, confusion, and alienation to the height of joy, fulfillment, and oneness with all of creation. The feeling area is that area through which we experience life. Most people believe (or allow) that their feelings are determined by the outside world. Such an attitude disempowers and makes one a passive receiver of very non-objective experience. A continuous emotional state of peacefulness and balance comes about as a result of opening oneself up to the divine grace that is all around us, always, ready for the taking. The physical act of breathing both reflects our condition in this area and can be adjusted in such a way as to learn to take in (be inspired) and give out (inspire others). Negative emotional states originate within us, have detrimental effects on our breathing, and then lead to problems in various physical parts related to breathing: the mouth, neck, throat; the bronchi and lungs, the chest, spine, abdomen, and even the lower extremities. A movement toward health is signified by deeper and more rhythmic breathing, as well as by a trend toward positive emotional states, inspiration, joy, and gratitude. In childbirth the spirit faculty is extremely important. Breathing is the metronome of inspiration that accompanies the melody of labor.

Hierarchical organization of the person

By examining a person's morphology we gain insight into all other characteristics of the person. The body's distinct expressions reflect non-visible tendencies and strivings of the soul. Most of what we see was present in the person's latent physical expression since life in the womb. Some of what we see has been acquired through habits accumulated over the years as physical or emotional compensatory mechanisms, or the result of suppression by drugs, crises, and emotions.

The three levels of being human are absolutely interrelated and connected in space and time. That is to say that anything influencing one aspect influences all aspects (space), and that every significant influence experienced at a point in time creates reactions on all of the three human levels, which continue to exert influence (i.e., compensation reactions), sometimes for a person's entire life. What's more, often these compensation reactions continue into the next generations (especially if they are not resolved in the current one). These are expressions of the vital force (see below) attempting to bring about equilibrium.

Each person (and indeed every being) is supported by what is termed the *vital force:* a force which works in us at all times to maintain homeostasis and allow us to remain among the living. It is that force which gives rise to our every symptom (whether pathological or simply descriptive). Therefore we say in homeopathy that symptoms are the expression of the vital force. We can know the vital force only through the symptoms it manifests. It brings about symptoms in the person as a means to maintain balance, or homeostasis. The vital force always acts on us in such a way so as to manifest symptoms on the most benign level possible under the given circumstances. The vital force cannot be quantified (that would refer to vital energy, which has ebb and flow depending on such factors as age, lifestyle, diet, stress, illness, etc.). Rather, it is a *force*. It works in us just as it did from the moment of our conception and goes on working until the moment of our death. Given a stimulus according to the law of similars, such as a homeopathic medicine, a person's vital force will react, in some way, until the moment of death. It reacts in the context of the myriad of constraints and blocks we put in its path: poor eating and lifestyle, medications which suppress and manipulate its action, emotional suppression, and so on. Some call this force the "wisdom of the organism." It is the force within every living being that causes change to occur. Its ultimate purpose is the maintenance of life as spiritually and physically productive and healthy as possible. The vital force is always dynamic: it is continuously reacting, because life is equivalent with movement.

The vital force can be observed on every level of creation: on the level of an individual being (mineral, plant, animal, human), and on the level of groups, humankind as a whole, or all of the created world as a totality. Every expression manifested by the vital force represents the realization of inner potential.

One's attitude toward the vital force and the symptoms it manifests determines how one will react when sickness or symptoms appear. Many people in the modern world—and most physicians—view symptoms as a sort of evil needing to be done away with. This attitude leads to suppression of symptoms, which has detrimental effects. Most people ultimately fear death, and therefore often unconsciously deny its existence, or do anything possible to make symptoms go away so as to not be reminded of death. There is a misguided assumption that illness is always a sign of pathology which leads to destruction of the person and—if not suppressed—death. The homeopathic view teaches that defining an illness as either good or bad is a moot point; illness, and the symptoms of which they are composed, manifest as merely the best possible viable option available to the vital force at the time, needed to keep the person in balance. The vital force can only act in the optimal way possible with what it has as constraints. No matter what it manifests as symptoms, its action is always a reflection of the whole and always acts on the whole. The whole does not leave anything out. It includes each level of the human being: physical body, emotional and mental spheres, and each part and level within each of those parts and levels. Then it is pertinent to remember that the person does not live in a vacuum but in a family, a group, a society, a country, a world, a planet in a solar system, occupying a particular place in the hierarchy of creation as a human being, having specific relationships with all levels of creation below this level (mineral, plant, animal) and above it (angels, archangels, and the entire celestial hierarchy up to God). Ultimately (many believe), every person is part of the Body of Christ. That is a more "holistic" holism. What this means in relation to the manifestations of the vital force is that symptoms (the vital force's language) both reflect and change a Whole that includes all of being. Therefore, suppression of symptoms changes the entire whole as well, and further initiates different reactions from the vital force.

Modern science is only now beginning to grasp, on its own terms, the tip of the holistic iceberg. The investigation into the human microbiome is changing medicine and philosophy of life. "Microbiome" is a collective term for all of the micro-organisms belonging to the three domains of bacteria, archaea, and eukaryota, while the "biome" comprises all life on earth. The microbiome is estimated to represent more than half of the total living matter (biomass) on the planet. What have been regarded as dangerous and bad micro-organisms, and provided the foundation for a trillion-dollar pharmaceutical industry for over 100 years, is now shifting: micro-organisms are now being acknowledged for having more than just pathogenic effects, and are being recognized as essential in the maintenance of life itself. Phages, for example, or the viruses that infect bacteria, are extremely important. Phages are the primary regulator of bacterial populations in the ocean, and likely in every other ecosystem on the planet. If viruses suddenly disappeared, some bacterial populations would likely explode; others might be outcompeted and stop growing completely. This would be especially problematic in the ocean, where more than 90% of all living material, by weight, is microbial. Those microbes produce about half the oxygen on the planet – a process enabled by viruses. These viruses kill about 20% of all oceanic microbes, and about 50% of all oceanic bacteria, each day. By culling microbes, viruses ensure that oxygen-producing plankton have enough nutrients to undertake high rates of photosynthesis, ultimately sustaining much of life on Earth.[7] Viruses are thus now understood as being vital in recycling materials. The processes being observed in the microscopic world are also the vital force at work.

Scientists acknowledge the all-encompassing influence the microbiome has on all of nature and for humans; it remains for them to equally acknowledge the effects that human beings exert on the planetary microbiome by suppressing symptoms within themselves with medicines and vaccines. Every action creates a reaction. The "war" so often referred to when discussing dreaded diseases is not a war between "innocent victims" and "evil pathogens," but, from the holistic homeopathic viewpoint, a war being waged by humankind against the vital force. If the vital force manifests itself in a pandemic disease, it means that this particular disease is the best possible solution at this point in time, for this particular organism (in this case, humankind as a whole). This is an enormously important philosophical issue. Its interpretation has massive consequences for humankind and for all of creation. The argument that mass vaccination will eliminate a pandemic is not scientific fact, but propaganda, sung to a fear-

---

7   Rachel Nuwer. (2020). "Why the world needs viruses to function." *BBC Future.* Available at: https://www.bbc.com/future/article/20200617-what-if-all-viruses-disappeared.

stricken public with virtually no opportunity for debate. The pandemic is regarded as some alien phenomenon that appeared out of nowhere, had nothing to do with any of us, and will disappear into nowhere once we have enough vaccinated individuals. There is no account of a vital force, of a purpose in anything, of our own participation in the life we observe in and around us. There is no attitude of *presence* with ourselves as a group. We allow ourselves to occupy the role of victims in a haphazard, accidental existence in which things happen *to* us.

The multi-level understanding of the person means that the vital force works on all levels at various times, and homeopathy has shown that where it will bring about symptoms at any given time can be relatively determined. In other words, there are objective laws that give us hints about what to expect. The levels of the person are hierarchical, with the mind being the deepest and most fundamental, and the physical body being the most superficial. The early 20th-century homeopath Constantine Hering discovered the most profound law of healing and illness: the vital force always works on the most surface level possible to bring about equilibrium. The most superficial level is that of the physical body. Within the physical body the skin is the most superficial part. But if the symptoms on the physical level are suppressed (by medications, emotions, outer conditions), then the vital force expresses itself on the next deepest level—the emotional level. If that level is also inaccessible, due to suppressive influences, then only the level of the mind remains.

Hering's law also demonstrates how one heals: from the deeper level to the more surface level, from the inside out. This means that surface-level acute illnesses usually involve the emotions or the thoughts only in a limited way, but if these illnesses are suppressed with drugs, the symptoms disappear on the surface level and the illness goes deeper to express itself either emotionally or mentally.

Symptoms are manifested by the vital force and they do not recede on their own until and unless they are "brought to fruition." This is a very appropriate expression when applied to the vital force and the symptoms it manifests. A fruit cannot drop from the tree until it is ripe. Each symptom has to be expressed to its specific fullness before it can wane, like a fever ever climbing until at some point it reaches its zenith, and then falls. Nobody can determine the exact temperature at which critical mass will be reached in a given person with a given illness. We can only say with certainty that this is the way of symptoms: they need to be fulfilled to their individual "logical conclusion." It is this understanding that is at the basis of giving a homeopathic medicine. The homeopathic remedy, prepared from a natural substance that causes symptoms similar to the ill person, is given in the most minuscule quantity, a minimum number of times, in order to assist the vital force in bringing symptoms to fruition more efficiently and quickly. By taking a substance in the most minimal amount possible (and most homeopaths prescribe micro potencies), the vital force is given just the slightest "nudge" in the direction in which it was already working, thus assisting fruition to be reached more quickly and efficiently.

Suppression of symptoms (acute or chronic illnesses; emotions; reproductive functions including operative delivery, abortion, anesthetized childbirth; hormonal contraception; etc) leads to the perpetuation of symptoms and patterns. It leads to chronicity and incurability. "What is inside must come out." On the one hand we have our vital force continuously working to maintain balance and harmony on all levels of our being; on the other hand, this force is often thwarted. Suppression of symptoms is almost always harmful (with the exception of suppression in order to save a life, for example during a hemorrhage), because it prevents the vital force's action to maintain homeostasis. Over time, if suppression continues, the vital force transfers its outlet of symptom-expression to a deeper level of the person. Every expression of the vital force (i.e., illness, event) is connected to every other expression. And so there is no such thing as random expression of the vital force. Everything it does is in consistence with natural laws. It expresses itself through symptoms that are characteristic of the person's particular miasm and constitution.

Constitution is a term used in classical homeopathy to refer to a person's symptom-totality as a whole. It includes the physical characteristics, likes and dislikes, characteristic reactions both physical and psychological, as well as predisposition to specific chronic problems and psychological patterns. A person's constitution changes over the course of a lifetime, in response to external influences, but most people don't sway too far from the constitution of their childhood.

The concept of *miasms* in homeopathy is similar to the idea of inherited tendencies in genetics. Miasms make up broader categories than constitutions (there is a limited number of miasms, whereas there are dozens of constitutional types). This concept is discussed in more detail later.

These basic concepts form the foundation on which it becomes possible to not only determine a person's morphological type, but also to understand how morphology, constitution, and miasms are connected. The homeopathic phenomenological view of the person helps us to become more accepting, forgiving, and loving—of those who are different from us, and with our loved ones. It puts into perspective our power (or lack of it) to change people and situations. We come to understand that although we can't change most things, we might be able to influence a person's process: their births, their self-awareness and self-acceptance, their ability to be fully present, their ability to speak and be heard, and their ultimate actualization.

For example, let's say we have a young woman, age 21, with a tendency toward weak muscles. She is average in height. Her hair is light brown and straight. Her skin is pale and her features fine. Her bones are thin, which is apparent by looking at the thickness of her wrists. She has had scoliosis since age seven, which her mother attributed to her "poor posture." She has flat feet, lacks energy, has no appetite, and seems to be far too thin to be capable of carrying a pregnancy to term. The same woman, applying as a student to acting school, loves theater yet is horrified by being on the stage and seems to be introverted in class. She rarely answers questions or contributes. Her voice is soft, weak, and inaudible. In this example we have the choice of analyzing each of her problems separately and then perhaps making disassociated recommendations or even sending her to several different specialists: she sees a chiropractor for her back issues, a nutritionist for her low weight and anemia, a psychotherapist for her stage fright, a midwife for her pregnancy, perhaps a voice coach as well. Our other option is interpreting her as a complete totality, a complete picture, in a holistic way through the help of homeopathic concepts. We can support the notion that no symptom happens accidentally but generally manifests itself as a defense mechanism; it is always part of a whole, which expresses itself in a hierarchical manner having the most vital aspect of the person at the center and the least vital aspect at the periphery. Our approach to facilitating growth and positive change in this young woman will reflect an understanding of that totality. In this example, we observe "lack of support," on every level: physically, emotionally, and mentally. This is nobody's "fault," but it does reflect the constitution—the predisposition—with which she was born. Her DNA is not "responsible" for her symptoms, but rather her symptoms (which were latent at her conception) are responsible for her DNA being the physical manifestation of an impulse of the vital force to bring her soul into incarnation in this specific way. This is *entelechy*[8] at work: the complete realization and final form of some potential concept or function; the conditions under which a potential thing becomes actualized. This particular woman already had *latent* stage fright, *potential* anemia, low weight, thin bones, and scoliosis at the moment of her conception. The vital force in her mother and father had prepared the way (completely non-consciously, of course) for the appearance of just such a person with these particular predispositions, because they (and several generations before them) had left much "unsettled business" in their bringing-to-fruition of their symptoms.

This idea of actualization, of making *explicate* what might be called *implicate intent*[9], might just change the way we regard symptoms, illnesses, morphologies, and of course other people. It changes the way we practice. When we acknowledge implicate intent (called by some "the divine plan"), we adopt a respect for its necessity. We stop trying to abolish

---

8   Entelechy, (from Greek *entelecheia*), in philosophy, that which realizes or makes actual what is otherwise merely potential.
9   Bohm, David, *Wholeness and the Implicate Order* (London: Routledge, 1980).

symptoms just for the sake of abolishing them (and our own life experiences). We start thinking about their actualization, their fulfillment, and begin to think creatively about how to best facilitate that actualization. Life can then be understood as a teleological process: an ever-becoming. This is different from suppression of symptoms! This is homeopathic understanding: that the actualization of tendencies can only be achieved by the law of similars. We want to always (whenever possible) move a person in the direction of the symptoms, ever so gently intensifying them through the homeopathic remedy.

Our gaunt, anemic future actress who is afraid of the stage and has trouble finding her natural voice, and whom we now encounter pregnant and nervous, will be helped first and foremost by an acknowledgment of her total condition. Our first "action" is always "do nothing." Dr. Robert Mendelsohn, with whom I became acquainted just after the birth of my first child and who became our family pediatrician, taught me this. We usually act out of fear when we see someone ailing. If only for a few seconds, the first thing we need to learn to do is: stop. Take a breath. Later I came to understand that this action is equivalent to acceptance of the person's symptoms and condition, or the person as a whole. Our pregnant woman is frail, anemic, and scoliotic because she does not assimilate minerals well. Her personality type indicates the psoric miasm—whose goal is survival. She has "survival" issues, as seen in her nutritional deficits and incapacity to speak. She lives for the most part in "first circle"[10], turned in toward herself. World-renowned voice coach Patsy Rodenburg coined the term "second circle" and defines it as: the optimal state between the first circle of introversion and self-doubt and the third of aggression and narcissism. In second circle a person is present, self-confident, and comfortable interacting with the world. Having acknowledged our woman's being for what it is, we support her through applying the law of similars; homeopathic constitutional treatment is in order which will not be aimed at bombarding her with supplements, but at prescribing a remedy that covers her case as a totality. Her remedy will be similar to her,

---

10   See Rodenburg, Patsy, *The Second Circle* (New York: W.W. Norton, 2008).

in that it induces symptoms similar to hers on every level, if taken in large doses by a healthy person. When she takes it however, the information in the remedy will find resonance with the information of the patient, there will be a mild intensification of symptoms, and then resolution will begin. The vital force will have gotten an extra, infinitesimal boost to achieve its strivings more easily. She will start absorbing nutrients from her food more effectively. She will feel more energy and a newfound sense of confidence. Her ribcage will expand with lower and deeper breathing. She will feel happier and somehow changed, although putting her finger on how and why will prove challenging. The positive effects will be passed on to her fetus, thus solving certain specific unresolved issues that might have otherwise been carried over to the next generation.

One's morphology is predetermined. That is, the body type of a child is obviously inherited from both parents and from previous generations. The specific expression of a morphological type is only relatively influenced by external factors during the mother's pregnancy: quality and quantity of food; lifestyle; physical exercise; climate; environment; sleep; her positive or negative habits; etc. It is important to understand the distinctions between natural selection and entelechy. Natural selection demonstrates that if certain traits are so malignant as to not allow a woman to get pregnant and give birth to a child—and thus to pass the traits on to her children—eventually, such traits disappear from the family branch. Entelechy demonstrates that significant symptoms that have been deeply suppressed in one generation will reappear in the next—if "allowed" by natural selection. The development of modern medicine since the end of the 19th century has had a massive influence on natural selection. Thanks to modern pharmaceuticals and operative childbirth, women who would have otherwise never conceived naturally, or who might have died in childbirth, and babies who would have otherwise not been born, now occupy an ever-growing percentage of human populations. Limiting the observation to pelvic type and shape in relation to its "passenger," we know that evolutionally less adaptive morphological types have become more prevalent in the last 100 or so years. With a holistic understanding of the relation between morphology (which starts with the pelvis) and every other aspect of human existence, we can also imagine that lots of other traits have become more prevalent in the human population as well. It's not only the pelvic shape that is passed down! Human beings of the third millennium see more predisposition to chronic disease, autoimmune and chromosomal abnormalities, cancer, psychiatric illnesses, and a host of other disease entities. Moreover, certain maladaptive personality traits and tendencies are more common.

When we look at a person's morphology, we are looking at symptoms: symptoms that needed expression, actualization. No symptom can be taken in isolation from the rest of the person, and no person can be taken in isolation from the preceding generations. The expression of symptoms now point to the likelihood that they were not adequately brought to fruition in previous generations. This is certainly true of serious chronic illness.

If the ability to be present, to be attentive and poised in one's environment, with one another, and with oneself, if the very predisposition to love was formerly a prerequisite for survival (and for reproduction), that trait, too, has become less prevalent in human society. Presence and love are no longer required either for sex or for reproduction. To our great sadness, they are no longer required to parent. In modern societies people seem to need each other less and less. This is as much a cause of our technological gadget-age as it is a result of it. What this all adds up to for those of us who are in the work of healing (of which theater is no less a part than midwifery or homeopathy) is the need to intensify our awareness. We are called to become continually more present ourselves, because all human beings everywhere need that presence more than ever.

CHAPTER TWO.

The Center of Morphology: The Pelvis

The study of human morphology could theoretically begin anywhere, but years of personal observation has taught midwives that it begins with the pelvis. The shape, size, and bone mass of the pelvis either determines or reflects every other part of the human form. Midwives in previous eras had a limited knowledge of how morphological differences were related to the course of labor and birth. Midwifery was traditionally the domain of women and was not open to study as a medical art for at least 16 centuries, following the dissolution of the Byzantine empire and ancient Greek medicine and until the consciousness change in Europe in the early 18th century. Various reasons are given for this historical fact, but whatever the explanation, it reflected a certain indifference to matters of women and childbirth, and amounted to neglect. Not surprising, then, that midwives in Europe were often historically regarded with a certain disdain. They were anything but indifferent to the fate of a laboring mother and her child and therefore were continuously searching for knowledge and skills that would aid them in their work. And any experienced midwife did know things. But women with knowledge—especially "secret" knowledge—were not always taken seriously by men, in a society which did not regard childbirth as a valid healthcare specialty. Detailed study of pelvic types was initiated with the appearance of the first lying-in hospitals in France, Germany, and Russia in the 18th century.

The most well-recognized classification system of the female pelvis in the West was developed by obstetricians William Caldwell (1880–1943) and Howard Moloy (1903–1953). Their system identifies four major types (gynecoid, android, anthropoid, platypelloid) and mixtures of these four. In classifying a woman's pelvis they looked at the sacrum, coccyx, sidewalls, sacrosciatic notch, ischial spines, pubic arch, and ischial tuberosities. In mixed types, the system requires placing the classification of the posterior portion first, followed by that of the anterior pelvis, separated by a hyphen, for example "android-gynecoid". Midwives and obstetricians used this classification system mostly in the first half of the 20th century for determining true disproportion. Before cesarean sections became extremely safe, it was necessary to be more careful and attentive in determining cephalopelvic disproportion and the need for operative delivery. After the 1950s, however, physicians started becoming less concerned about ensuring vaginal birth commensurate with the safety of operative birth, and the rate of cesarean delivery started to rise exponentially. Simultaneously, performing pelvimetry became more symbolic than practical. The art of pelvimetry was pretty much thrown out by obstetricians and midwives alike, the proverbial baby with the bathwater, but with it went the nuances that once fueled the passion of facilitating birth.

Russia, on the other hand, has a different obstetrical history: together with France and Germany, Russia was elemental in the birth of *classical midwifery* at the end of the 18th century, when Catherine the Great ordered the construction of the first maternity hospital in St. Petersburg to serve the needy and the sick. The maternity hospital became a place where midwifery could be studied as a medical art. Consciousness was changing; those in academic and religious circles now acknowledged the acceptability of intervening in childbirth with the purpose of saving the mother and child, in contradiction to the previous attitude of "The Lord giveth and the Lord taketh away."

Russian midwives and obstetricians continued using their own classical methods for pelvic classification, and still apply them, to a limited degree, to this day. In the West, however, the pelvis and its relation to the mechanism of labor was being formulated in the early 20th century.

The three Ps

The Scottish obstetrician John Martin Munro Kerr, professor of midwifery at the University of Glasgow from 1927 to 1934, determined six factors that influence the course of labor of every woman:

1. The form and size of the pelvis.
2. The flexibility of the pelvis.
3. The degree of rigidity of the cervix.
4. The size, position, and flexion of the baby's head.
5. The moldability of the baby's skull.
6. The effectiveness of the uterine contractions.

Each factor is related to one of three elements of the childbirth process, which Kerr called "the three Ps": passage, passenger, and powers. This system of understanding factors influencing labor is still applied to this day. Later, birth attendants added the fourth "P"—psyche: the psychological state of the woman, in particular the primipara, which may influence the course of labor.

Passage	Passenger	Powers
Form and shape of the pelvis	The size, position, and flexion of the baby's head	The effectiveness of the uterine contractions
The flexibility of the pelvis	The moldability of the baby's skull	
The degree of rigidity of the cervix		

The Pelvis

In midwifery reference is made to both the pelvis and to the *pelvic cavity*. The pelvis refers to the actual bones of the entire structure, whereas the pelvic cavity refers to the space bounded by the pelvic bones. If birthing a baby is our concern, it is the *space* that interests us most, and the quality of this space is determined by the material boundaries. Space is interesting for more than just midwifery purposes: space is where a person finds and from whence a person uses the breath, which then becomes the foundation on which the voice is used.

The pelvic cavity is home to the reproductive organs, as well as the bladder, the colon, and the rectum. The latter is at the back of the pelvic cavity, toward the sacrum and coccyx, whereas the bladder sits behind the pubic symphysis. A host of blood vessels and nerves are crowded into this space as well. Trouble with one organ or vessel or nerve has an influence on the other organs, vessels, and nerves of the space. The pelvic floor (or pelvic diaphragm) comprises the area underneath the bones of the pelvis and the pelvic cavity, forming a "bowl" which cradles the contents of the pelvic cavity. Both men and women have conscious control over the muscles of the pelvic floor. We tighten them under tension (or when we need to use the toilet but can't get there fast enough). The pelvic floor plays an enormously important role in self-awareness, freedom of expression, and self-esteem. It is directly related to our breathing patterns; chronic pelvic floor tension leads to breathing high up in the chest. It is also related to the degree of tension in the throat. Women who tend to get a lump in the throat as an emotional reaction also tend to have pelvic floor tension. A closed or tense throat is associated with prolonged dilation of the cervix in the labor of primiparous women. These tendencies also are connected with unsatisfactory intimate relationships, and an inability to trust and be present.

The pelvis is composed of three parts: two innominate bones (what we are accustomed to calling the hip bones), the sacrum, and the coccyx. They are connected from birth by cartilage and begin the process of ossification in the womb, which continues in a relative fashion into early adulthood.[11]

---

11   Alik Huseynov, Christoph P. E. Zollikofer, Walter Coudyzer, Dominic Gascho, Christian Kellenberger, Ricarda Hinzpeter, and Marcia S. Ponce de León. (2016). "Developmental evidence for obstetric adaptation of the human female pelvis." *PNAS.* 113(19)5227-5232.

Female pelvis

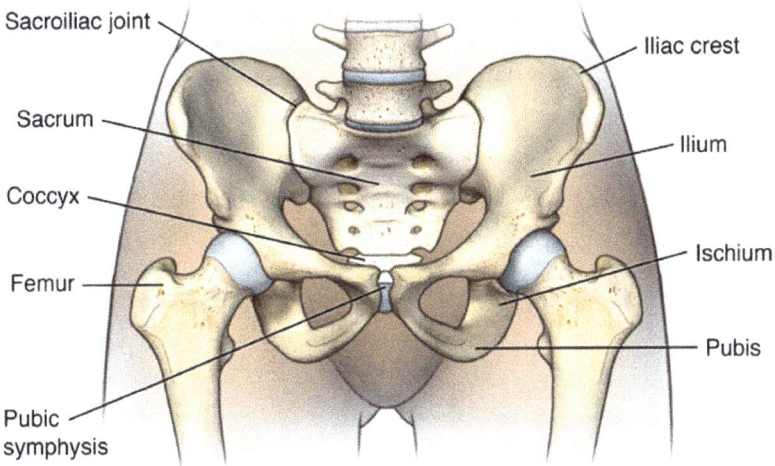

Sacroiliac joint

Sacrum

Coccyx

Femur

Pubic
symphysis

Iliac crest

Ilium

Ischium

Pubis

1. **Innominate bones** consist of three separate bones:
   - **Ilium** (there are two, one on each side; in the plural we say **ilia**): the large bones on the top of the pelvis that form the point that sticks out on either side; the part on which a mother props a baby);
   - **Ischium** (also two; plural = **ischia**): makes up the lower posterior third of the pelvis; the branches compose the open corner in the front and the "sits bones" underneath. In the posterior border of the bottom of the ischium (or what we consider the mid pelvis from the inside) we meet a triangular eminence on either side, called the ischial spines. The diameter between them constitutes the transverse diameter of the mid-pelvis: also known in midwifery as the "plane of least dimensions," because it is usually the smallest diameter in the false pelvis and, traditionally, the deciding one—which makes the difference between a physiological vaginal birth and an operative delivery.
   - **Pubic symphysis**: compromises the anterior wall of the pelvis. The upper and lower branches of the pelvis are connected here by cartilage, in a relatively inflexible union. This area often becomes painful at the end of pregnancy as the baby puts pressure on it,

especially in multiparous women. The location of the pubic symphysis relative to the pelvic floor provides a lot of information about the shape of the woman's pelvis, as well as the angle of the pelvis in relation to the spine. A pelvis that is more tipped, at a smaller angle relative to the ground, exhibits what looks like a "lower" pubic symphysis (and a more rounded, defined bottom), whereas a pelvis sitting at a greater angle relative to the ground seems "higher" on the lower abdomen, and the woman's bottom is much flatter.

2. **Sacrum**: a large triangular bone at the base of the spine, which forms after sacral vertebrae S1 to S5 fuse between the ages of 18 and 30. It is nested between the ilia at the back. The sacrum forms joints with 4 bones: with the ilia on either side (creating the sacroiliac joints); with the last lumbar vertebrae (L5) at the top; and with the coccyx at the bottom. The sacrum is generally concave (to a greater or lesser degree depending on one's morphology). The uppermost part of the sacrum is tilted forward to create what is internally discovered as the sacral promontory. This projection into the upper part of the lesser pelvis creates the posterior border of the pelvic brim— the first pelvic plane the baby enters as it prepares for birth. The sacrum (or *holy bone*) is considered historically and universally the most significant bone in the body, all the more for our purposes; therefore it is discussed in detail in a separate chapter.

3. **The coccyx**: the lowermost part of the human spinal column, composed of four or five fused vertebrae. It connects to the sacrum at the sacral-coccygeal joint. It is usually mobile, but may not be so, if the person suffered trauma.

The pelvis as passage

Obstetricians first started documenting the connection between difficult childbirth and pelvic shape and size in the 16th century. Henry Van Deventer was called the "father of the pelvic theory" in 1701. By the middle of the 18th century, knowledge of the female pelvic proportions and the fetal skull were mandatory parts of practicing the new medical specialty of obstetrics, especially owing to the popularity of the obstetric forceps. William Smellie (1697–1763), the renowned man-midwife known as "the father of British midwifery"[12], contributed to the knowledge of the physiology of childbirth possibly more than any other person in the modern medical era. Smellie was highly respected as a teacher as well as a midwife. His students did not gain any certification or fulfill medical training requirements by attending his courses, but came seeking to enhance their knowledge. As a teacher, Smellie tried to provide his students with live demonstrations to go along with course lectures. Consequently, he offered free midwifing services to patients if they allowed his students to observe the birthing process.

The bony pelvis serves as a rigid passage through which the baby must pass. The general size and shape of the pelvis directly influence the course of labor. The cervix and vagina are soft tissues, which make up the birth canal and also contribute to how the baby will move through the passage, but they have a relative influence. The specificities of the pelvis are of interest to us, be we practitioners of any sort or women or men, because they give us hints about the totality of the morphological type, which in turn gives us information about the person as a whole.

The flared upper part of the bony pelvis is called the greater (or *false*) pelvis, and it is not considered part of the bony passage. That part of the pelvis, located lower than the *linea terminalis*, is called the lesser (or *true*) pelvis. It is the true pelvis that is of relevance to midwifery.

12   Smellie, William, *Treatise on the Theory and Practice of Midwifery*. Ed. with annotations, by Alfred H. McClintock (London: The New Syndenham Society, 1876).

The pelvic planes and the curve of Carus

Authors have delineated three, sometimes four, planes through which the baby must travel on its way out of the womb. They are divided into separate planes owing to the curve of the pelvic cavity. This is known as the curve of Carus, and it has an approximately 90-degree angle from the pelvic brim to the pelvic outlet. When standing, the pelvis slopes into a position where the pubis is lower than the sacral promontory—described as an angle of 45–55° to the horizontal or to the floor. This slope continues throughout the cavity, reducing its angle to 15° at the outlet. The fetal head is required to negotiate its way through the curve of the pelvic angles. It enters the brim in a downward and backward direction and undergoes a spiral rotation as it moves toward the pelvic floor.

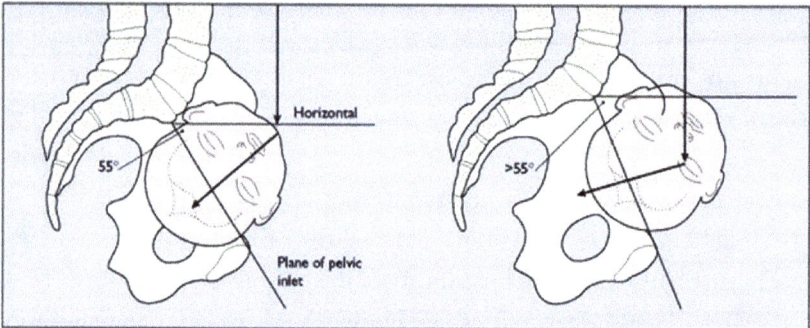

The baby enters the pelvis at the brim at a 55-degree angle relative to the ground. In the picture on the right, the pelvis is tilted forward, making the angle much greater and increasing the difficulty in descent.

A nuance such as the **tilt of the pelvis** is for the most part morphologically (i.e., constitutionally and miasmatically) determined. Different morphological types have different degrees of pelvic tilt. A woman's living habits have only a relative influence on the degree of pelvic tilt, because it is generally determined morphologically and is related to the bony structure. Sedentary lifestyles, years of carrying babies on their hips or in a sling, and breastfeeding can influence the tendency toward an anterior pelvic tilt temporarily. Wearing tight-fitting jeans and walking in high-heeled shoes throughout adolescence influences the pelvic tilt more significantly during a period of growth before the pelvic bones have ossified. However, just as scoliosis or lordosis is not simply a result of "bad posture," anterior or posterior pelvic tilting is not the result of unhealthy living habits, unless of course a person has suffered severe malnutrition. The morphological category is determined even before the embryonic stage of a person's life. It is a given at the moment of the creation of the soul. It is as much a part of the person as the form of the oak tree is to the oak. Morphology is a reflection of the soul's individual and unique journey—the journey appropriate to that particular human being with the benevolent intent of the vital force.

The pelvic tilt influences the center of gravity: pelvic types displaying a deep, funnel-shaped pelvis (such as the android type) force the breath upward together with the center of gravity (and the baby during pregnancy). Interestingly, this "male pelvis" (another term for android morphology) displays the highest center of gravity, which is characteristic of men. The pelvic tilt also determines the "natural" level of the correctly placed breath low in the abdomen. This level is not identical between morphological types, although the spectrum is narrow and it requires much practice in morphology in order to determine an individual's "natural" level of the lowered and placed breath.

The planes

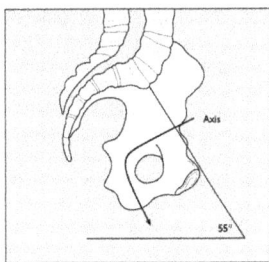

The curve of Carus. The pelvic planes and their varying angles from inlet to outlet.

The pelvic planes include the inlet, the mid-pelvis (or cavity) and the outlet. The Caldwell-Moloy classification system was concerned at the time (i.e., early 20th century) primarily with the size and shape of the inlet. This is explained by the fact that at that time, cesarean deliveries were avoided due to potential risks involved. It was generally accepted that if the baby could descend into the inlet, it could be born; whether it was born alive or dead was secondary, since the risk of operating was significant to the mother.

Later, with the increasing safety of cesareans, this attitude was replaced by a new approach: if modern medicine was now capable of saving just about any baby who would have otherwise died due to cephalopelvic disproportion without risking the mother's life, it followed that the mid-pelvis and the outlet became more interesting areas of study, since the new goal became not just getting a baby through a pelvis—live or dead—but birthing live babies.

For midwives and especially in the home-birth setting, the value of determining a pregnant woman's morphology in making a prognosis about her labor cannot be overestimated. The assessment gives the midwife and the mother an idea about what to expect during a first labor and birth, and therefore helps in the prevention of potential complications because proactive recommendations can be made.

Knowing that the tilt of the pelvis varies relative to the overall morphology of the woman, we can make approximate predictions about other things; for example, if the tilt is greater than average (i.e., anterior pelvic tilt), as in the anthropoid morphology, the woman is more likely to carry her baby outwardly; her longitudinal abdominal muscles are more likely to be overstretched, with possible diastasis in a multiparous woman; the baby might take longer to descend into the inlet in a multigravida; and the vertical position for this woman could have the effect of weakening contractions, since it reduces pressure from the baby's head on the cervix. These are the type of women who experience more effective contractions lying on their side. A woman with a less than average pelvic tilt (i.e., posterior pelvic tilt), on the other hand, has a problem similar to the first one in that it is not an optimal angle for the baby's easy descent into the inlet. This is observed with the android morphology. But in such a case, the woman carries her baby "high" and "inside." The baby tends to lie in the occiput-posterior position (i.e., occiput toward the posterior part of the mother's pelvis) and the head "rides" on the pubic symphysis. The posterior pelvic tilt is evidenced by the woman's seemingly "high" pubic bone in the supine position, and flat bottom, with a low buttocks crease. Such women tend to choose the hands-and-knees position during labor.

Modern theory asserts that 1) pelvic tilt is caused, for the most part, by poor posture and habits; 2) anything other than neutral pelvic tilt is perpetuated and/or caused by "tight" or "weak" muscles, ligaments, and fascia, which are themselves caused by posture and habit; and in conclusion, that 3) these problems are created by the person herself albeit subconsciously, and can be corrected through exercises. For example, one author explains:

> Anterior pelvic tilt is caused by the shortening of the hip flexors, and the lengthening of the hip extensors. This leads to an increased curvature of the lower spine, and of the upper back. Posterior pelvic tilt is the opposite of anterior pelvic tilt. It occurs when the pelvis rotates backward, causing the front to rise and the back to drop. It is caused by lengthening of the hip flexors and shortening of the hip extensors.[13]

Such assertions run contrary to the homeopathic understanding of the person, which places **implicate intent** of the vital force at the center. This driving mechanism has only one purpose: the maximum actualization of the soul. What we see are the particular ways in which the vital force works toward this actualization. These ways can be classified into groups of similar forms and patterns. Secondly, such assumptions neglect the reality (and necessity) of individuality as expressed in diversity. There is no one ideal form—nor one ideal pelvic tilt angle—but only variation within a spectrum, each of which expresses the intention of the same vital force to move toward restoring the soul's divine image in which it was created. Nature is known for her biological diversity: the variability among living organisms on the earth, including the variability within and between species and within and between ecosystems. Biodiversity is the variation of life at all levels of biological organization, referring not only to the sum total of life forms across an area, but also to the range of differences between those forms. Biodiversity runs the gamut from the genetic diversity in a single population to the variety of ecosystems across the globe. Biologists assert that:

---

13   Leonard, Jane. (2017). "Six fixes for anterior pelvic tilt." Available at: https://www.medicalnewstoday.com/articles/317379

Greater biodiversity in ecosystems, species, and individuals leads to greater stability. For example, species with high genetic diversity and many populations that are adapted to a wide variety of conditions are more likely to be able to weather disturbances, disease, and climate change. Greater biodiversity also enriches us with more varieties of foods and medicines. Beyond its intrinsic value, biodiversity is necessary to human survival. Ecosystem diversity is crucial to ecosystem integrity, which in turn enables our life support, giving us a livable climate, breathable air, and drinkable water. Food-crop diversity and pollinating insects and bats allow agriculture to support our populations; when disease strikes a food crop, only diversity can save the system from collapse. Plant and animal diversity provide building blocks for medicine, both current and potential; almost half of the pharmaceuticals used in the United States today are manufactured using natural compounds, many of which cannot be synthesized. They also provide critical industrial products used to build our homes and businesses, from wood and rubber to the fuels that underpin our economies—even coal and oil are the products of ancient plant matter and preserved zooplankton remains.

Biodiversity plays a central mythic and symbolic role in our language, religion, literature, art, and music, making it a key component of human culture with benefits to society that have not been quantified but are clearly vast. From our earliest prehistory, people have never lived in a world with low biodiversity. We've always been dependent on a varied and rich natural environment for both our physical survival and our psychological and spiritual health. As extinctions multiply, and cannot be undone, we tread further and further into unexplored terrain—a journey from which there is no return.[14]

---

14   "The Elements of Biodiversity." Center for Biological Diversity. Available at: https://www.biologicaldiversity.org/programs/biodiversity/elements_of_biodiversity/

In our anti-diversity age we are challenged to not only embrace variation but to study it and learn from it. Diversity—of opinions, experience, values, indeed cognition as a whole—is itself under threat of extinction. As holistic inquirers we ask, "Where is this going, and how?" rather than "What caused this phenomenon and how can I change it?" The "cause" is always the same: the vital force helping the soul toward equilibrium and actualization. The "where" and the "how" are the specific clues we will use to help the person reach this equilibrium via the law of similars.

The inlet

Each of the three pelvic planes has at least four diameters: the anteroposterior (front to back); the transverse (side to side); and the oblique (from one corner to the opposite corner, on both sides). The fifth important diameter is the posterior sagittal diameter, usually only taken into account in the mid-pelvis. As the baby makes its way through the pelvis,

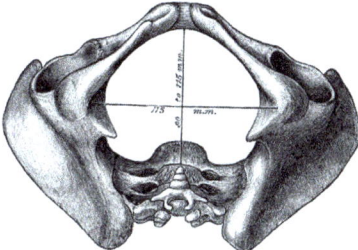

The transverse and anteroposterior diameters of the inlet from below.

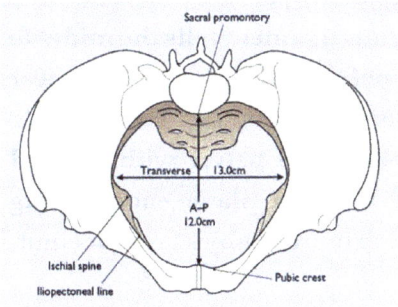

The inlet from above.

it does so in a fashion similar to the DNA helix: in a spiral motion. Usually the baby descends into the inlet with the sagittal suture of the head in the transverse diameter, parallel to the transverse diameter of the pelvis. This is because the longer occipitofrontal diameter usually finds the best fit into the wider transverse diameter of the inlet of the average woman's pelvis. When the head descends in another diameter of the inlet, it is because it can, i.e., the fetal head always occupies the path of least resistance.

The midpelvis

The midpelvis is the most significant of all the planes in our age of modern medicine because it is considered the "plane of least dimensions." The least of the diameters of this plane is usually the transverse diameter. It is also wonderfully fascinating that women have been created in such a way that this least of the pelvic diameters is given to us via reflexive expression in the rhombus of Michaelis, where we find it revealed in its exact measurement. If a midwife were given only one element about a woman's morphology in order to make a prognosis about her birth, this would be the information she needed, even if it meant forsaking all the rest: and she could discover it merely by looking at, and palpating, the woman's rhombus.

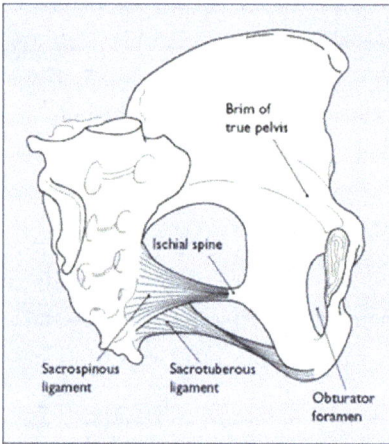

Cutaway of the midpelvis.

The ischial spine marks one side of the transverse diameter. It is generally masked by the sacrospinous ligament and therefore not obvious on internal examination. Its quick and easy identification on the other hand indicates a morphology type other than gynecoid. The examiner knows when she's found the spine during an internal exam because the examinee reacts with a sudden noise (the pudendal nerve runs alongside the ischial spine).

The width of the sacrotuberous ligament tells the midwife about the degree to which the pelvis converges in the lower portion. A short sacrotuberous ligament and encroaching ischial spines indicate a funnel-shaped pelvis with a small posterior sagittal diameter of the mid plane—not leaving much room in the posterior section for the baby's large occiput.

The outlet

The outlet of the pelvis has its borders on the coccyx in the back, the pubic symphysis in the front, the ischial tuberosities on each side. Since it is generally longer from front to back than wide, by the time the baby gets down to the pelvic floor the head has no choice except for the long axis to rotate into the anteroposterior diameter. In most cases this *internal rotation* (one of the steps in the mechanism of labor) occurs as the baby's head descends onto the pelvic floor and completes its turn within just one or two contractions. With the succeeding contractions the head, rather than flexing, starts deflexing and extending until it gradually begins to dilate the vaginal opening and can be seen between the labia.

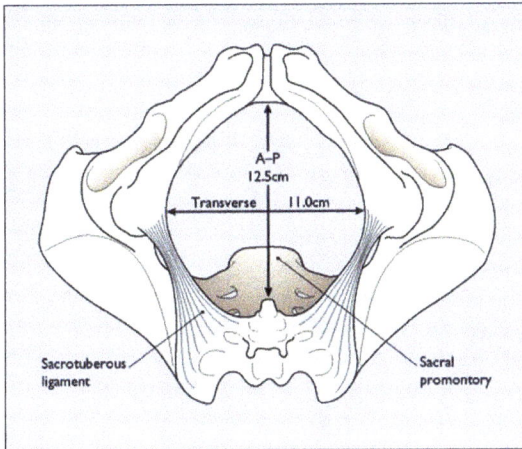

The pelvic outlet. From this angle it is easy to see how the shape and size of the outlet is related to the placement of the acetabulae in the hip sockets, which consequently influences how the legs balance the person's weight and their relation to each other.

The outlet tells us what will happen when the baby's head navigates its exit from the birth canal. The minimal required transverse diameter, which falls between the "sits bones," is 10 cm. Anything narrower than that—assuming the baby's head is at least average size—causes the head to slow its descent, as well as forcing the head posteriorly toward the rectum. This can result in lacerations of the perineum and potentially the anal sphincter, especially in a fast birth. Sitting in a squat widens the transverse diameter of the outlet, but should only be undertaken when the head is already on the pelvic floor and about to emerge, since the squatting position also narrows the transverse diameter of the inlet.

A wide transverse outlet presupposes a tendency toward the platypelloid morphology, with its general transverse width and antero-posterior reduction. This could mean the baby descends in the oblique diameter and never completes internal rotation into the anteroposte-rior diameter—as it doesn't need to. Sometimes the head is even born in the transverse diameter. Additionally, a short anteroposterior diameter could predispose to shoulder dystocia in a large baby. The midwife's awareness of the woman's morphological specifics helps her to predict potential nuances in delivery.

CHAPTER THREE.

The Morphological Assessment

Classical (external) pelvimetry method

Classical pelvimetry requires the use of a pelvimeter. Knowledge about the female pelvis was initiated by the French obstetrician Andre Levre (1703–1780). He was the one who invented the terms "inlet" and "outlet," identified the oblique diameters of the pelvis, introduced the concept of "minor pelvic axis," and developed the basic model of the classical obstetric forceps. But the greatest service to classical pelvimetry was made by the outstanding 18th-century French obstetrician Jean Louis Bodeloc (1746–1810). He developed and improved the methods of English obstetrician William Smellie (1697–1763), who introduced the measurement of the pelvis into everyday obstetric practice and described in detail the flat-horizontal pelvis (since rickets was common in Europe at that time), and corrected many mistakes typical of his time. He is known for introducing obstetrics in France to the rank of scientific discipline. He wrote a comprehensive work, *The Principles of Midwifery*, which for many years became the main textbook on the midwifery art for doctors and midwives around the world. It was Bodeloc who created the pelvimeter: an anthropometric caliper for measuring external dimensions of the pelvis. He proved that bone deformity of the internal pelvis can be detected through its external dimension. The external means of measuring the pelvic inlet, or *conjugata externa*, was called the "Bodeloc diameter."

Later, it was suggested that this external feature is inferior to the internal dimensions of the inlet according to the Smellie method, i.e., *diagonal conjugate*. In Western Europe the *conjugata externa* has not been used since the 1950s, while all pregnant women in Russian women's clinics are still being measured to this day.

The external method is simpler and less intrusive for women. The internal method of assessing the diagonal conjugate is relevant only if the practitioner is using this one measurement as the sole criterion for assessing the pelvis—an absurd proposition. In addition to the external measurements (all, and not just one), the amount of space in the true pelvis can be assessed by determining the woman's bone mass (using the Soloviev index, for example; discussed later).

Although pelvimetry is used traditionally for the sole purpose of determining pelvic adequacy, it has a wider application for midwives and others interested in more: it can tell us not only the means by which a baby will likely be born, but the likely character of the labor itself. Pelvimetry allows us to determine pelvic classification as well as general pelvic volume within a particular classification. It tells how a labor is likely to progress in every phase.

Mastering external pelvimetry is handy for the student who will be eventually attending births. It is convenient, in that it can be performed without uncomfortable intimate exams. It does not increase the risk of infection to the pregnant woman because no internal examination is performed. Additionally, it can be performed during labor very quickly—in situations where the midwife is seeing the woman for the first time—and efficiently without seriously disturbing the laboring mother. It is a good academic exercise, although it can be completely superseded by examining the rhombus of Michaelis and other key elements of a woman's morphology in order to come to an understanding of the whole.

Diameters of the female pelvis, determined using external pelvimetry

The measurements given for each diameter represent the average for a gynecoid pelvis. Accordingly, any deviations from the average are indicative of a different pelvic type. All of the measurements obtained from external pelvimetry are reflections of the approximate internal diameters. Although both historically and in modern times pelvimetry is regarded separately from all other morphological characteristics, it is in fact of no value if taken in isolation. The morphological method is all-inclusive and holistic; pelvimetry on its own is not.

The Four Diameters

1. *Distantia cristarum*: the distance between the most distant points of the iliac crests. The average diameter is 28–29 cm. This size corresponds with the width (transverse diameter) of the pelvic inlet. The diameter is taken into account in relation to the other measurements.

2. *Distantia spinarum*: the distance between the anterior superior points of the ilia. The average size is 25–26 cm. This size gives us an approximate idea of the thickness of the bones, if considered in relation to *distantia cristarum*. A large difference between these two sizes (more than 3 cm) indicates thick bone mass and a smaller volume of the false pelvis.

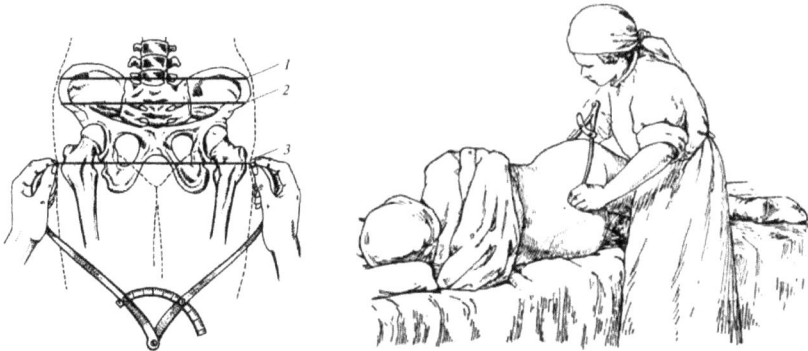

The diameters of external pelvimetry: 1) distantia cristarum, 2) distantia spinarum, 3) distantia trochanterica, and on the right: measuring the conjugata externa (drawings from old Russian obstetric textbook).

3. *Distantia trochanterica*: the distance between the large balls of the trochanteric femurs in the widest dimension. The average size is 31–32 cm. This value reflects the transverse diameter of the pelvic outlet and the degree of its general narrowing. A diameter less than 30 cm with a wide *distantia cristarum*, for example, indicates a funnel-shaped pelvis and potential problems with fetal descent.

4. *Conjugata externa* (Bodeloc diameter): the distance between the upper part of the pubic bone and the upper edge of the sacrum. The average size is 20–21 cm. This value reflects the anteroposterior diameter of the pelvic inlet. In order to approximate the diameter of the *conjugate vera* (true conjugate, or the actual diameter inside the pelvic brim minus the bones), 9 cm are subtracted from the external conjugate. If the woman is determined to have thin bones based on her Soloviev index (measurement of the wrist circumference) of 14 cm or less, then 8 cm are subtracted from the external conjugate rather than 9. Similarly, if her wrist index is 16 cm or more, she has massive bones, and 10 cm are then subtracted from the external conjugate.

The diagnosis of contracted pelvis is traditionally made on the basis of the small size of the *conjugata externa*. Using external pelvimetry, it is impossible to determine the volume of the pelvis on the basis of the size of only one diameter because other sizes can compensate for contracture. The dimensions per se are not absolute without considering the woman's bone mass, overall size of the pelvic cavity and its relation to the size of the presenting part of the baby, its position and the mobility of the cranial bones (determined by gestational age).

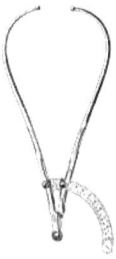

A pelvimeter

In Europe and the US, the pelvimeter went out of fashion in the 1950s, as external pelvimetry was rejected in favor of internal, and then internal was all but abandoned. In the West the art of pelvimetry itself has been lost, and external indicators have lost their significance. This has occurred in connection with the progressive medicalization of childbirth, loss of clinical skills in favor of technology, and the trend toward more intervention and cesarean sections. Medicalization, in turn, came about

The Morphological Assessment

in great part due to pressure on obstetricians from insurance companies who could not afford to have suits brought against hospitals or doctors when birth outcomes were less than optimal. Such trends in medicine have all but eliminated the need for and interest in numerous classical clinical[15] methods for practice. Practitioners who retain the passion for analysis, for making deductions and prognoses based on clinical observations, find their interest squelched and their inquiring minds thwarted by technological domination. The practice of looking first to ultrasounds, monitors, and laboratory analyses has led to a pathetic loss of skill (if skill was ever acquired in the first place) and the overall lowering the bar of medical practice standards. This phenomenon is probably more applicable to obstetrics than to any other medical field, and the proof of it lies in the disproportionately high operative and interventive delivery rates throughout the world, rates that do not correlate with lowered morbidity and mortality for mothers and babies.

Modern (internal) pelvimetry method

In the 18th century, William Smellie developed a method by which it is possible to better determine the direct size of the pelvic inlet. The diameter is called the diagonal conjugate (*conjugata diagonalis*). This value shows the distance from the lower edge of the symphysis to the most prominent point of the sacral promontory. The diagonal conjugate is determined by internal vaginal examination. The second and third fingers are inserted into the vagina, the fourth and fifth fingers are bent, and they rest against the perineum. The fingers inserted into the vagina are directed toward the sacral promontory, and the edge of the palm rests on the lower edge of the symphysis. After this, the second finger of the other hand marks the place of contact of the examining hand with the lower edge of the symphysis. Without lifting the finger of the second hand from the marked

---

15 "Clinical" means those procedures and methods of analysis that require the use of all sensory organs—sight, smell, hearing, touch—for making prognoses. Clinical skills, for example, are contrasted with test results.

point, the fingers located in the vagina are removed and measured in centimeters (with the help of another person). The measurement of the diagonal conjugate is then the distance from the top of the third finger to the point of contact with the lower edge of the symphysis. For the great majority of women (and depending on the size of the examiner's hand) the sacral promontory is impossible to reach. The diagonal conjugate of a normal pelvis is an average of 12.5–13 cm. To determine the true conjugate, 1.5–2 cm are subtracted from the size of the diagonal conjugate.

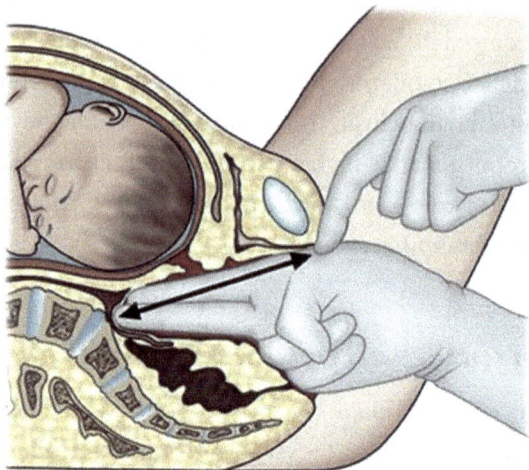

Measuring the length of the diagonal conjugate based on the length of the examiner's fingers. Note that the measurement is possible only if the examiner's fingers reach the sacral promontory (which happens very rarely in women with normal pelves when examined by midwives, most of whom are women, whose hands are not always large).

In the 20th century, internal pelvimetry expanded to include new characteristics:

- *Symphysis inclination.* The longitudinal axis of the symphysis is usually parallel to the longitudinal axis of the sacrum. If the symphysis is not at least approximately parallel to the sacrum, the direct size of the entrance changes significantly.
- *Angle of the pubic arch.* The descending branches of the ischia and the lower edge of the symphysis form what is called the pubic arch. The angle of this arch should be at least 90°, as defined, just below the symphysis.

The Morphological Assessment

- *The general structure of the anterior pelvis.* The arch of the anterior pelvis should be rounded. An anterior pelvis with a more square shape reduces the oblique dimensions of the entrance.
- *Lateral pelvic wall angles.* The lateral walls of the pelvis usually tilt slightly toward each other, but they seem parallel on vaginal examination. Sharply converging walls indicate a decrease in the size of the pelvic outlet and the angle of the pubic arch.
- *Sacrosciatic notch.* The shape and width of the sacrosciatic notch are important in that they affect the posterior sagittal diameter of the inlet, which forms, together with the shape and curve of the sacrum, a space for the baby to pass in the normally roomy posterior portion of the pelvis.

It is helpful to understand certain moments from the history of obstetrics in order to put the application of pelvimetry into perspective. By 1938 in the United States, half of the births were taking place in hospitals. This increased to 99% by 1955. By the 1970s, the percentage of home births once again started increasing as more women started seeking natural birth. Cesarean sections became relatively safe—and therefore more and more common—in direct reflection of this trend. Before the 1940s, doctors had a more serious clinical interest in determining a woman's prognosis for labor before labor began. Pelvimetry was useful not only for assessing pelvic adequacy per se, but also in assessing the potential risk of forceps delivery. As cesarian section became safer, the number of forceps deliveries decreased—at first doctors abandoned "high" forceps, and gradually started avoiding the application of mid-forceps.

Another new technology to be discovered in the early 20th century was radiography. Obstetricians were overjoyed to be able to use X-rays for determining things like gestational age, fetal position, placenta previa, anomalies, etc. Radiography was also used extensively as a method of pelvimetry. It was used from 1924 until approximately 1975—more than 50 years!—before the medical world became convinced that its risks outweighed the dangers of its use. By that time, alternative methods of imaging had been devised which are far less dangerous.

The clinical vs. technological camps, apparently, were formed from the very beginning. A practitioner's allegiance to one or the other is not determined so much by their gender, title, level of formal medical education, or intelligence, but by a foundational attitude toward childbirth itself: is it merely a means to the end of producing a child, or is it an essential basic experience with ontological significance for women? If a practitioner adheres to the latter interpretation, then her role includes doing whatever possible to assist a woman to give birth as naturally as possible and in such a way that the woman is able to be completely present to the experience. As for internal pelvimetry's value for the contemporary practitioner, all of these landmarks and their significance have their place in the totality and therefore they shouldn't be shunned as superfluous. Rather, they should be regarded for what they are: relative. What we seek to identify is the totality of a particular and unique woman, the whole always being more than the sum of its parts. The totality can be identified by just a couple of symptoms, if those symptoms are sufficiently characteristic.

Morphological characteristics

Height. A person's height is considered genetic, but homeopaths have observed that height is also connected with the dominant miasm in the individual and in the family. Ethnic variations aside, we find that tallness is most commonly associated with the tubercular miasm. From the homeopathic repertory of symptoms we find the rubric **Generalities; tall** to contain the following remedy substances[16]: *arg CALC CALC-P carb-v guai*

---

16   The homeopathic repertory of symptoms is a reference containing all possible symptoms in the form of "rubrics" (a shortened way of describing a symptom in a person). The remedy substances given for a particular rubric indicate that those substances are capable of producing such a symptom as part of the group of their pathogenetic symptoms. Remedy substances are always abbreviated according to a universal system of abbreviation. Remedies in a lower case font are capable of producing the given symptom to a mild degree; those in italics are a bit more likely to produce the symptom; those that are capitalized are very likely to produce the symptom, and when both capitalized and in italics, the strongest likelihood of all is indicated.

IOD kali-c kreos MAG-P PHOS SEC sulph thuj tub. In this group of remedies, being tall and large-framed is more characteristic of Calcarea carbonicum, Kali carbonicum, Sulphur, and Thuja—and, as would have it, those remedies have more of a tendency toward android and android-gynecoid morphologies. Among short people we encounter all of the miasmatic nosodes except for the Psoric nosode, Psorinum: (***Generalities; dwarfishness****: ambr aster bac* **BAR-C** *bar-i BAR-M bor CALC* **CALC-P** *CARBN-S carc CON iod lyc mag-m MED merc merc-pr-a nat-m nep OL-J op ph-ac phos pitu-gl sec SIL sulfa* **SULPH SYPH** *thyr TUB zinc.*). Here it is noteworthy that Syphilinum, the nosode of the Syphilitic miasm, is expressed in the strongest degree. Assessing height in absence of general morphological characteristics is of course one-sided. We can arrive at a holistic picture only after taking all elements into account.

It is traditionally believed that a woman shorter than 150 cm has little chance of giving birth naturally. However, the average height of a woman from a pygmy tribe in Central Africa is no more than 5 feet (155 cm), despite the average weight of a newborn pygmy being 8 pounds (3600 g). This suggests that the size and shape of their pelves are quite sufficient for natural childbirth. Height does not necessarily indicate small pelvic size. In addition, adults of short stature are not born small, just as a large infant with heavy birthweight and longer than average length is not necessarily destined to become a tall adult. However, the normal diameters of the rhombus are constant and universal for women of all statures—that is, the **minimum required 10 cm transverse diameter between the dimples of the rhombus applies, whether a woman is 6 feet tall or 5 feet tall.**

Bone mass. In addition to evaluating the rhombus, the midwife measures the circumference of the wrist, the so-called Soloviev index. This indicates the total thickness of the bones and averages 14–16 cm. A wrist circumference more than 16 cm means that the woman has massive bones and, accordingly, less space in the small pelvis. Paradoxically, the smallest and thinnest women have the thinnest bones, like a porcelain doll, and give birth very well, insofar as they have more space in the false pelvis. Bone mass informs us not only about family tendencies toward such a frame but also about the "structural" aspect of a person in general. A person with massive bones naturally has more structural substance in the physical body and more micro-elements of which bone is composed. If we ponder the question from the standpoint of compensation, we might venture to say that building a strong house for oneself on earth is a compensation for the desire for safety, security, stability, predictability (Psora)—or, possibly, a "building-up" or amassing of substance, an accumulation of material strength, a statement of "I am here!" (Sycosis). Small bone mass displays a different tendency. We say that thin-boned people are like birds, who can be blown away by the wind. Such a morphological characteristic reflects an issue around the micro-elements of structure (calcium, phosphorus, silica, etc.) and their assimilation, and also suggests an ethereal, not-of-this-world image.

Legs. The morphology of the legs—their relationship to each other, shape from top to bottom—reflects the relationship, first and foremost, between the femoroacetabular joint and the acetabulum (in absence of any malnutrition diseases, genetic syndromes, or other conditions that influence leg shape). The femoroacetabular joint is a *ball-and-socket joint* that joins the femoral head to the acetabulum.

The ball-and-socket articulation allows for a high degree of mobility. In comparison to the shoulder joint, it permits less range of movement due to the increased depth and contact area, but displays far more stability. The acetabular labrum increases the depth of the joint. The joint is surrounded by a fibrous capsule, which is attached to the acetabulum, and then attaches to the proximal aspect of the femur. Thickenings of this capsule constitute the ischiofemoral, iliofemoral, and pubofemoral ligaments.

In order to clarify the morphological type, we examine the legs and notes their overall shape and gaps when the legs are placed together at the feet. The shape from hip to heel indicates the presence of such characteristics as *internal rotation of the legs at the hip* (which is seen as knees coming together or knock-knees); *external rotation of the leg from the hip* (which presents as knees not touching when standing with feet together);

pronation (the weight of the leg is on the inside of the foot) or *supination* (the weight of the leg is on the outside of the foot).

- Gynecoid people have the classic Marilyn Monroe three-gap leg shape: a gap between the thighs, under the knees, and above the ankles.
- Android morphology: "knock-knees" or x-shaped legs. The thighs touch from the hip to the knee and then the legs deviate outward away from each other. The person cannot stand with feet together without bending one knee to accommodate. Morphologically determined knock knees can be distinguished from rachitic knock knees (*genu valgum*), the latter of which are associated with malabsorption of calcium and phosphorus constitutionally; however, rickets is more often expressed as *genu varum*, or bowed legs.
- Anthropoid morphology: the legs are straight as a tree trunk from hip to heel. They are close together and usually come into contact with each other all the way down.
- Platypelloid morphology: there is a space between the legs from the hip down to the feet and the knees don't touch each other.

The leg shape clearly begins with the pelvis, and reflects such individual characteristics as:

1. The ball-and-socket articulation itself (depth of the acetabular labrum);

2. Overall diameters of the pelvis: the transverse diameter adds or subtracts from the leg width;

3. The overall depth of the pelvis: a longer, deeper pelvis tends toward more shallow hip sockets, while a shorter pelvis tends toward more roomy ones;

4. Shape of the pelvis from above: influences the degree of rotation in order for the legs to maintain stability.

Feet. The size of the foot (i.e., footwear) shows only random correlation with ability to deliver vaginally, although that said, proportional measurements of all physical characteristics speak in favor of natural birth. The length of the toes and width of the foot corresponds, naturally, with the overall morphology. A platypelloid morphology includes a wide foot and relatively short toes. An anthropoid morphology expresses the opposite: long toes and a narrow foot.

Forearm length. We are interested in the length of the forearms as a predictive factor in childbirth: we can assume a favorable outcome for childbirth in a woman if the length of her forearm is no less than 42 cm from the tip of the middle finger to the elbow. A shorter length indicates overall pelvis contraction.

Hyperlaxity of extremities. The location of the arms in relation to the waist during active walking indicates the presence or absence of joint hypermobility. This characteristic is called in folk language "bucket-carrying capacity." Elbows that brush the waist reflect hyperlaxity of the joints, and display the same almost inverted shape as the x-shaped legs, which themselves reflect hyperlaxity. Taken together with other features it is possible to assess the morphological type and also to make certain prognoses. This trait most often corresponds with android morphology and heavy bone mass and potentially reduced capacity inside the lesser pelvis. It also indicates potential problem areas during pregnancy (back pain from compensatory muscle spasm), symphysitis with extreme separation of the symphysis). See chapter on android morphology for detailed description of joint hypermobility.

Fingers. The length and shape of the fingers also reflect the general morphology. Fingers that are extremely short and square correspond with heavier bones and smaller dimensions. Extra-long, tapering, and narrow fingers correspond with women who are taller, and narrower in the transverse diameter of their bodies, and wider in the anteroposterior diameter (anthropoid).

Head shape. The general shape of the woman's head also corresponds to the shape of the pelvis and oftentimes speaks of the necessary proportions that nature gives to the woman and her baby in labor so that the latter can pass through the pelvis. It only makes sense that the head shape reflects the pelvic shape and that the fetus will have at least some degree of similarity to the morphology of its mother and father. Variation, naturally, has come from ethnic diversity.

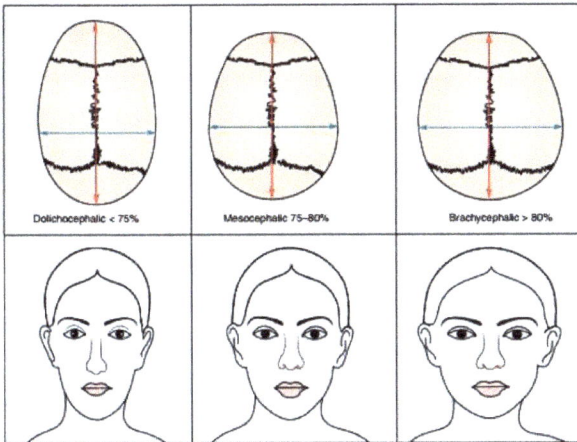

Cephalic index and head shape. There undoubtedly exist far more than three shapes. It can be postulated that the shape of the occiput mirrors the shape of the inside of the sacrum.

The concept of cephalic index was introduced in the 19th century as a means of classifying races based on head shape and indicates the percentage of breadth to length in any skull. The index is calculated from measurement of the diameters of the skull. The length of the skull is the distance from the glabella (the midpoint between the brows) and the most projecting point at the back of the head. The breadth of the skull is the distance between the most projecting points at the sides of the head, usually a little above and behind the ears. The cephalic index is the breadth multiplied by 100 divided by the length. An index of less than 75 means that the skull is long and narrow when seen from the top; such skulls are called dolichocephalic and are typical of Australian aborigines and native[17] southern Africans. An index of 75 to 80 means that the skull is nearly oval; such skulls are called *mesocephalic* and are typical of Europeans and the Chinese. A skull having an index of over 80 is broad and short, and is called *brachycephalic*; such skulls are common among Mongolians and the Andaman Islanders. Some 19th century scientists tried to prove the association between cephalic index and intelligence. This association was never proven. The value of observing head shape lies in seeing its correspondence with pelvic shape and overall morphological type.

---

17   The Editors of Encyclopaedia Britannica. (2011). "Cephalic index." Encyclopaedia Britannica. Available at: https://www.britannica.com/science/cephalic-index.

Metopic Suture
The metopic suture, which runs along the midline of the frontal bone will fuse normally between the ages of three months and nine months.

Sagittal Suture
Full obliteration may never occur. The suture closes sometime between 30 and 40 years old. The suture has been seen to close normally at age 26 and also remain open until someone in their late 50s.

Coronal Sutures
The coronal sutures may begin to fuse by the age of 24. On average they close between the ages of 30 and 40.

Lambdoid Sutures
Full obliteration may never occur. The suture closes normally between the ages of 30 and 40.

Squamosal Sutures
Sutures close between 30 and 40 years of age.

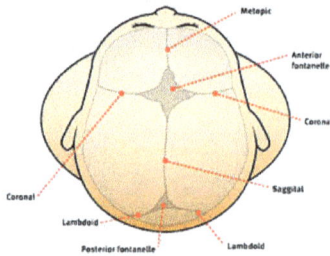

Frontal Sphenoid
May close normally by the age of three months.

It is only logical to assume that in a platypelloid morphology, for example, the head shape would mirror that of the pelvis; a flat occiput is more characteristic of Eastern peoples, and such a head easily engages in the transversely wide platypelloid pelvis. A flat occiput doesn't require a lot of space in the posterior part. And the opposite is true: people with a large occiput and a narrow face have a narrow transverse and long anteroposterior diameters—both of the cranium and the pelvis. The cranial bones fuse at their various sutures surprisingly late in life[18].

Face. The morphology of the face also reflects the morphology of the pelvis. A woman with a flat, wide face, and wide-set eyes has the same pelvic type: wide in the transverse, but flat in the anteroposterior diameter. High cheekbones with a square lower jaw often indicate a heart-shaped pelvis and thicker bone mass. The arch of the upper teeth, looked at from below, can also say a lot. The arch of the anterior teeth corresponds in shape to the anterior part of the pelvis. With a capacious pelvis, the teeth fit well in the mouth. Teeth that are misaligned and poorly fitting reflect pelvic contracture in one or more diameters. Such observations would only seem to be common sense.

---

18   "Skull Sutures—when do they close?" CAAPS Kids. Available at: https://www.cappskids.org/skull-sutures-when-do-they-close/

Respiration, the diaphragm and the infrasternal angle

Breathing is an enormously significant action of the body, well beyond its function of respiration. We know that breathing is the foundation for both voice and presence work. A well-placed breath determines our being heard and understood. It determines the quality of the voice. It is related to one's relationship with the world and one's willingness to "be inspired" as well as to "inspire" others. The most charismatic and inspiring individuals have a well-placed breath.

The diaphragm functions during breathing when it contracts to enlarge the thoracic cavity and reduce the intrathoracic pressure so that lungs may expand and fill their alveoli with air. In the thorax it is called the thoracic diaphragm and serves as an important anatomical landmark that separates the thorax, or chest, from the abdomen. It is a dome-shaped muscle and tendon that functions as the main muscle of respiration and is essential to the breathing process. It is a fibromuscular sheet that has a convex upper surface that forms the floor of the thoracic cavity and a concave undersurface to form the roof of the abdominal cavity. The esophagus, phrenic, and vagus nerves, descending aorta, and inferior vena cava pass through the diaphragm between the thoracic and abdominal cavities. The diaphragm is asymmetric with the left side slightly more inferior than the right, chiefly because of the presence of the liver located on the right. The left side may also be partially inferiorly located because of the push by the heart[19].

The diaphragm is the motor muscle of breath, which can be automatic, forced, or controlled. The diaphragm is assigned to multiple functions, both indirectly and directly, which go beyond breathing. It also promotes expectoration, vomiting, defecation, urination, swallowing, and phonation. The diaphragm influences the body metabolic balance and stimulates the venous and lymphatic return, thereby creating the correct

---

19   Oliver KA, Ashurst JV. (Updated 2021). "Anatomy, Thorax, Phrenic Nerves." *StatPearls* [Internet]. *Treasure Island* (FL). Available from: https://www.ncbi.nlm.nih.gov/books/NBK513325/

relationship between the stomach and the esophagus to prevent gastro-esophageal reflux. It is essential for correct posture and locomotion, as well as for the movement of the upper limbs. The diaphragmatic muscle influences the emotional and psychological spheres. Inspiratory apnea is able to raise the somatic pain threshold, decreasing the painful perception[20]. How one's diaphragm is used relates to many things, not the least of which is the individual morphology of the person.

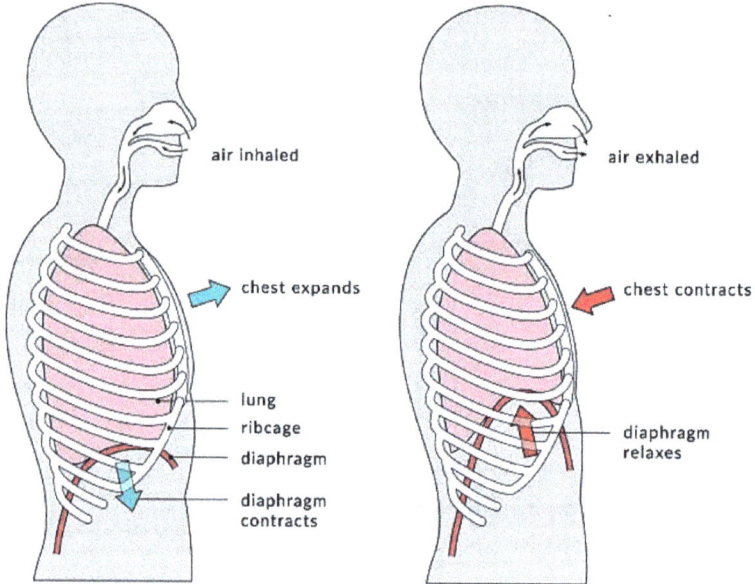

air inhaled

chest expands

lung
ribcage
diaphragm

diaphragm
contracts

air exhaled

chest contracts

diaphragm
relaxes

The **infrasternal angle** (ISA, or subcostal angle) is formed in front of the thoracic cage by the cartilages of the tenth, ninth, eighth, and seventh ribs, which ascend on either side, where the apex of which the xiphoid process projects. The average angle is 90 degrees. Anything wider is considered a wide infrasternal angle, and anything narrower is considered a narrow infrasternal angle. The ISA is a representation of an individual's respiratory strategy, that is, inhalation and exhalation, also commonly referred to as expansion and compression. A wide ISA creates

20   Bordoni B, Purgol S, Bizzarri A, Modica M, Morabito B. (2018). "The Influence of Breathing on the Central Nervous System." *Cureus*. 10(6):e2724.

The Morphological Assessment

a bias toward inhalation, meaning the person can inhale more effectively than exhale, whereas a narrow ISA creates a bias toward exhalation, meaning the person can exhale more effectively than inhale. A person can acquire unhealthful respiratory habits which may lead to over-dependence on auxiliary muscle support for breathing and speaking; this can result in all kinds of problems, including pain in various areas, vertebral issues, sleeping disturbances, digestive troubles, and so on. Although the ISA is not "to blame" per se, it is an element in an overall morphological picture. Like all morphological traits, the ISA hypothetically predisposes a person to specific adaptation strategies. It is only logical to assume that a person's diaphragm (shape, size, location) is also representative of the overall morphological type and therefore the way people use their diaphragms varies.

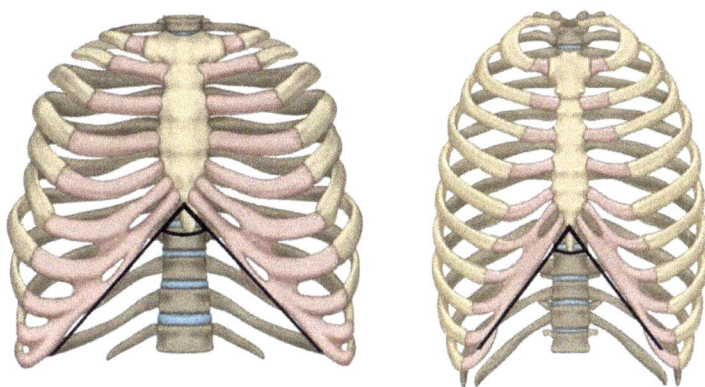

Infrasternal angles: wide (left) and narrow (right).

A wide ISA—considered by many to be 110 degrees or more—accompanies a relative flattening of the anteroposterior diameter, just as the pelvis does, while a narrow ISA—60 degrees or less—has a longer anteroposterior diameter. The ribcage on the right is compressed laterally compared to the ribcage on the left. This compression is a reduction of space and limits the person's ability to "expand" (increase the space) laterally as they breathe. The breathing in a narrow ISA directs more air anteriorly-posteriorly, not only because it's the path of least resistance but because it is what the thoracic cage allows, while the wide ISA is more compromised in the AP diameter but more advantaged laterally.

A wide IFA is more common in android morphology and in android-gynecoid combinations, in which we observe internal rotation of the tibia, femora, and pronation of the feet, with a simultaneous compensatory external rotation of the knees.

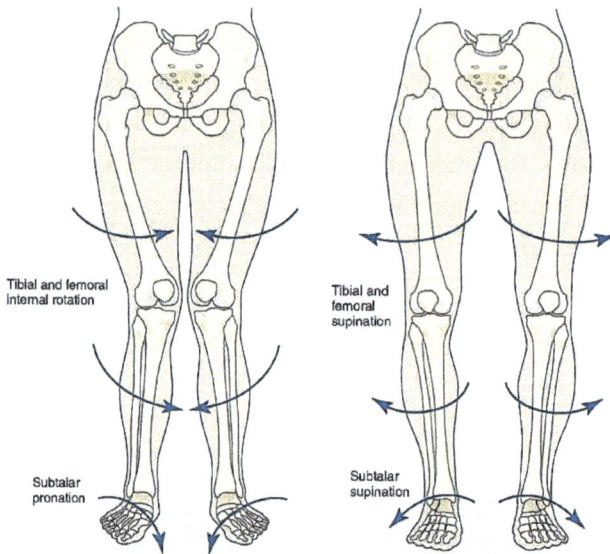

These morphological types tend toward lordosis of the spine as compensation for the top-heaviness and internal rotation of the shoulder girdle. Over time, if the compensations become extreme, they affect the breathing and subsequently the character and quality of the voice and the capacity for self-expression, which is often "locked" into a third-circle adaptive stance. This "locked" quality belies the very sensitive inner being of the person, whose adaptation responses reflect a need for stability and "grounding." This tendency is symbolized in the bias toward inhalation (taking in; and in its extreme form, avarice, covet-ousness), and weakness in exhalation (giving out; accepting; loving). Simple exercises for learning diaphragmatic breathing with an emphasis on slow, full exhalations can help such an individual find a more truly restorative means of adaptation which ultimately will lead to not only a more genuine, open voice, but also to more second-circle relationships of mutual trust.

A narrow IFA is more common in the anthropoid and anthropoid-gynecoid mix morphologies. In this case we observe a tendency toward external rotation of the tibia and femora and supination of the feet (putting the weight on the outer part of the sole)[21].

These tendencies are not necessarily observed in every person with a particular morphological type but point to areas of compensation. Practitioners of all specialties can gain insights into the observed nuances of their clients and then work with those compensations—including patterns of breath and its relation to how one holds the physical body on the earth.

21　(2021). "A Comprehensive Guide to the Infrasternal Angle & Compensation Layers." Pinnacle Performance. Available at: https://www.conorharris.com/blog/a-comprehensive-guide-to-the-infrasternal-angle-exercise-selection

The Morphological Assessment

Chapter four.

The Sacred Bone

The term *sacrum* in English derives from the Latin, *os sacrum*— literally "holy bone." The sacrum is a source of numerous mystical associations. The Latin term comes from the Greeks, who termed it the ἱερόν ὀστέον. Moderns speculate on why the ancients called the bone "holy"[22]: some consider it is related to the fact that the sacrum is the strongest bone in the body and the last to decompose after death. Others suggest that in Greek the word means not only holy but "temple," perhaps in reference to the sacrum enclosing the temple of the uterus, the source from which human life emerges. Still others propose that the sacrum is the energetic center of the physical body, the union point between heaven and earth. Gnostic writers attribute mystical significance to the sacrum, with its spade shape reminiscent of the grave-diggers' spade; it signifies both our mortality and our immortality. Following the trail through several explanatory hypotheses about the origins of the name sacrum, renowned neurosurgeon Oscar Sugar introduces evidence that the sacrum in tradition was the bone necessary for resurrection, identifying it as the "almond" or *luz* of the Hebrews and the *ajb* of the Arabs, and ultimately deriving its conceptual underpinnings from the ancient Egyptians.[23] Various occult groups believe that as the base of the spine, it is the beginning of the 33 vertebrae, the foundation of knowledge and eventual wisdom. In many

---

22   Ojumah, N., & Loukas, M. (2018). "The Intriguing History of the Term Sacrum." *The Spine Scholar* Vol 2, no.1.

23   Sugar O. How the Sacrum Got Its Name. *JAMA*. 1987;257(15):2061–2063.

holistic medical modalities the sacrum is known to be the energetic center from which treatment begins. Healing has to start at the core, otherwise one risks suppressing the symptoms. Stross puts forward an argument, using ethnographic, linguistic, and iconographic evidence, that the sacrum bone was a sacred bone, that it played a significant part in some Prehispanic Mesoamerican iconographic and cosmological traditions as it did in some Old World cultures, that it was related to reproduction, fertility, and reincarnation, and that in Mesoamerica the sacrum represented one index of the more generalized but variously manifested "portals" or doorways permitting translocation of shamans, spirits, and deities between worlds or levels of the cosmos.[24] Classical midwifery, too, corroborates this knowledge: the rhombus of Michaelis is visible and palpable on the external side of the sacrum and it represents the window to a woman's morphology and thus to her sacred birthing space.

Although the significance of this term is shrouded in mystery for the modern materialistic world, the Russian term for it reveals a post-Christian association: крестец (krestets) in Russian, or "small cross." Indeed, the four-sided rhombus of Michaelis, adorning the sacrum like a tablecloth, has the form of a cross. The top sagittal section is shorter, in the majority of women, than the longer lower section. Fascinating indeed, that Jesus lived 33 years—the quantity of vertebrae in the spinal column not including the sacrum—and ended His earthly human life on the cross, only to be resurrected. How marvelous that the ancients intuited, well before Christianity, that the cross of the sacrum is somehow representative of eternal life. This speaks to a deep knowledge about the holy bone that surpasses the explanations or "comfort stories" of the conscious mind. Some might posit that it also indicates divine prophecy in material form: even since before the birth of Jesus, His presence—parousia—was evident in the human form.

This reverence for the holy bone crossed cultures and oceans at a time when there was no communication, no physical contact between

---

24   Stross, Brian. *The Mesoamerican Sacrum Bone: Doorway to the Otherworld.* (University of Texas at Austin, 2007).

continents. It was a kind of innate knowledge common to diverse cultures in various epochs. Such universal understandings about our being and the various meanings our being has in all its expressions are innumerable. Unfortunately, this way of understanding the world, this inherent symbolic thinking which happens of its own accord when a person is totally present in the environment, has all but disappeared from modern culture. It has become almost impossible to comprehend with our hearts and in our bodies what we know personally and as societies. The rational mind suppresses the innate-irrational knowledge of the heart. We have lost nearly all of our symbolic-ritualistic acts that in a former age held us together, served as the mortar for the bricks of human culture. We have all but lost our stories. *Once upon a time, a long time ago…*we forgot what happened. It just happened that meaning has been lost. We have replaced, and continually replace, meaning with its cheap imitations. Tragically, we have stopped believing in almost everything. Symbols are no longer meaningful, or they are assigned random unshared meanings from the rational mind. We ourselves are *being* less and less. Where there is a paucity of meaning, there can eventually be no existence, because meaning *is* being. What we could formerly do in the way of symbolic acts on a subconscious level as an expression of *meaning* and therefore *being* in our lives, we have forgotten. We have a need however for living our meaning, for experiencing life as authentic, and so we observe many people creating spiritual-symbolic cosmologies for themselves, pieced together from odds and ends of random cultural remnants from cultures long extinct. Witness the myriad neo-pagan movements. People need symbol, meaning, culture—we need connection, an awareness and a surety of our place is the cosmos.

The ancient and unconscious knowledge about the sacrum has relevance because the sacrum is the center of the physical body, the top of the physical hierarchy holding the organism together as a whole unit, and therefore whatever is going on with the sacrum reflects what is going on with the entire person. This word "reflects" is very significant here, because one might attempt to say that uncovering an imbalance in the sacral area, and then balancing it, would be healing. This is essentially the assumption of chiropractors, osteopaths, and body workers. They take, for the most part, the imbalance as the problem itself, rather than seeing it as an outward expression of the "inner." In that case one asks: what is this "inner" that exhibits itself in the outer? As discussed previously, the inner is the soul, and therefore the physical symptoms we are capable of witnessing represent the soul embodied. We can term it thus: the sacrum's particular way of manifesting itself expresses the *tropos* of the soul. Its particular form, size, characteristics, and whatnot provide us with information, symptoms about the deepest part of the person. The essence is manifested in the form, and that is its *in-formation*. Knowing this—our attitude about "what to do" with the sacrum is altered.

Simply manipulating what we might interpret to be an imbalanced sacrum—making it balanced, as it were—would be suppressive. There is meaningful intent and purpose behind why a certain woman's rhombus looks the way it does. Knowing that the vital force works toward equilibrium in the most optimal way possible, we can also then know that this particular rhombus and this corresponding sacrum within this particular corresponding pelvis within this unique body—which is the earthly incarnation of an infinitely precious soul—came into being just as it was meant to, in fact only as it was possible to. All kinds of factors played a part in how and why this individual structure was manifested just as it was. Such factors include specific aspects of the implicate intent (enfolded potential) of the parents and grandparents that was unsolved in them, not brought to fruition, and therefore surges forward to be expressed in the next generation; also included is the degree of suppression of symptoms in the person in question, as well as in those who gave birth to her. Every soul has its goal as actualization, blossoming of what is inside, like the information in the acorn waiting to become a grand oak tree. This "bringing to fruit" is the nature of life. It is, itself, healing. And it is also meaning itself. *The extent to which a soul does not actualize during the earthly life corresponds proportionately to the depth of its despair and suffering.* That's not to say that actualization is not painful. But eliminating pain and suffering is not the goal of a true healer. Our goal is the same as that of the Orthodox Christians: to assist people, insofar as it is possible, to move as far as they can toward their own personal actualization of their divine *logos*, or defining principle from God, restoring the divine idea from which every person was created. We are now attempting to recover both the heart-knowledge itself and, even more vitally, the capacity for it.

The knowledge about the sacrum can be taken at face value. The world and the people who live in it display a hierarchical organization from bottom to top or from core to periphery, and on each level there is a central element holding that particular piece of the universe/person together. This is true of every level individually, and each level exhibits a certain similarity to each higher level.

Such phenomena speak to the idea proposed by quantum physicist David Bohm, that meaning *is* being, unfolded and revealed in form. This is expressed in the word *in-formation*:

> information is a very condensed form of meaning that has to be unfolded. Information by itself may be irrelevant or just wrong, but information is the form within, virtually. But obviously that form as the meaning is not complete without the whole meaning and all the contexts spreading indefinitely. So the concept of information is very limited without adding and bringing in the meaning…. Meaning is something like the form which informs the energy, so it will actively direct the energy and shape it…. Meaning organizes everything…. Mind and matter are inseparable, in the sense that everything is permeated with meaning. The whole idea of the somasignificant or signasomatic is that at no stage are mind and matter ever separated. There are different levels of mind. Even the electron is informed with a certain level of mind…. In so far as any meaning determines what it is, how it acts and so on, it is behaving in a way similar to how a mind acts….[25]

What we observe in the created world is the unfoldment, as Bohm called it, of an inner virtual potential. The form of the sacrum—or any other

---

25   Meaning as being in the implicate order", an interview from Basil Hiley, ed. *Quantum Implications: Essays in Honour of David Bohm.* (Routledge, 1991).

part of the body—is the expression, the manifestation of meaning. It is an intention, or an idea, crystallized. Orthodox Christian fathers and mothers of the Church might say that each person, and indeed every created being, is an expression of God's idea. God had an intention in creating any particular soul, and the body in its specificities is the physical embodiment of that soul and that intention. When we observe common expressions (like the quantity of vertebrae or the presence of the rhombus over the sacrum) it speaks to a common "road" (tropos) for humankind in a collective path to actualization of the divine idea. This can be applied to all parts of the body, but the sacral area/rhombus is clearly special insofar as it has been singled out as having a special relationship with birth, death, and eternal life. One might assert that it is the energetic center of the physical body. This has long been known in Asian and other traditional medical practice, however expressed differently.

It means, at the very least, that as practitioners of various kinds and simply

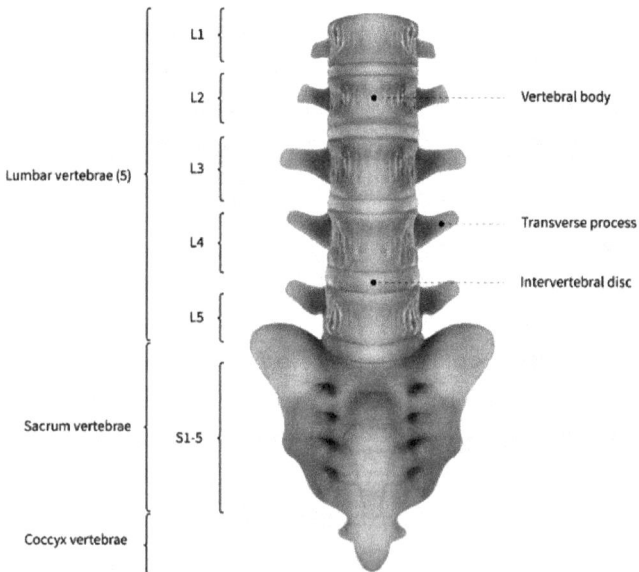

The lumbar vertebrae in relation to the sacrum

as observers or participants in our own *tropos*, we need to pay particular attention to the rhombus of Michaelis. It means that this area holds a key to the character of actualization (birth, life, death) of this person and therefore assists us in diagnoses and prognoses. For homeopaths it points to potential miasms and constitutional types. For midwives it gives hints as to what to expect during the birth, and tells us how we might work with the person for individual therapies. For voice work it tells us why a person is having trouble in a specific area, how it might be related to their breath and presence in their body. It is a constructive tool. It doesn't end with classification, and it is not limited to obstetric pelvimetry. And the point is not to make all holy bones conform to an ideal structure, but to use the knowledge gained from observation to lovingly respect individuality (and avoid the human desire to "perfect" it), assisting the person to work with their own nuances of form.

Pelvimetry tells us a lot about the overall size of the pelvis and the size of its individual parts and diameters. But the data obtained from pelvimetry is purely mechanical; they tell us about the probability of a baby being capable of fitting through a particular pelvis. They don't tell us about how the woman is likely to labor, what the chances are of her carrying a posterior baby, whether she is likely to have a large baby, or whether or not she is likely to have premature rupture of the membranes. Pelvimetry alone makes no allusion to a woman's likes and dislikes, her overall character, or her potential problem areas. Traditional pelvimetry should not be used separately from the totality of the woman. The genius and splendor of morphology lies in its revealing interconnectedness of the human person. One part or region of the person indicates another part or region. This phenomenon demonstrates the aggregate nature of the person. The whole is visible in its parts. The tree is known by its fruit. And the center of these hierarchically organized parts is the sacrum as revealed in the rhombus.

In addition to the rhombus of Michaelis, there are many other areas of the body that indicate the shape and size of the pelvis, but the rhombus does so instantly and completely. It reminds us of the sacred nature attributed to it as a portal to eternity. It is the explicate expression of God's idea about the person; not just expression, but meaning. The form indicates its meaning. According to the **doctrine of signatures,** dating from the time of Dioscorides and Galen, herbs resembling various parts of the body can be used to treat ailments of those body parts. Paracelsus (1493–1541) taught the concept, writing that "Nature marks each growth…according to its curative benefit." The writings of Jakob Böhme (1575–1624) developed the doctrine of signatures. He suggested that God marked objects with a sign, or "signature," for their purpose. Böhme's 1621 book *The Signature of All Things* gave its name to the doctrine. The sacred bone's appearance informs us about its meaning and place in humankind and in creation. Persons were created for eternal life. We don't need to know every single minute detail about the person in order to understand their potential pathological tendencies, positive traits, reproductive problems, relationship difficulties, or veritable dominant attitude toward the world! We can look first to the rhombus. After that, more clarifying questions become obvious for the purpose of differential diagnosis.

In homeopathy there is an excellent exercise for students during which they are asked to identify the "symptoms" of a lemon. After much study of the fruit, students compile a huge list of every possible symptom. Following this, they are asked to choose five or six random symptoms and relay them to a person over the phone and ask them to guess what they are describing. At the end of the exercise everyone understands that identifying a lemon requires only two symptoms—but the symptoms must be the most characteristic. The same is true for understanding a woman's morphology (which, in turn, helps us understand the woman as a whole). The human person, and all of creation, is organized hierarchically. We don't require an endless list of characteristics, lab tests, and diameters. We require only the essential information. We require only the rhombus of Michaelis—the little cross. "Then Jesus told his disciples, 'If anyone would come after me, let him deny himself and take up his cross and follow me'" (Matthew 16:24). The cross as a symbol represents not only the trials and tribulations which one must bear, but also—and perhaps more importantly—the path to actualization of the soul. Its individual and unique form in any particular human body is like a map of where to discover the buried treasure. It provides the general direction, which in turn implicates nuances of the journey.

Διάγνωση—diagnosis

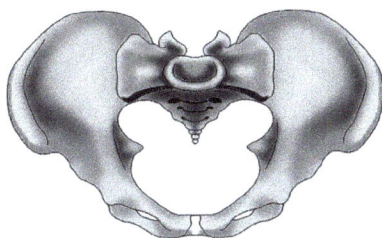

The shape of the inlet and its correspondence with the shape of the rhombus.

From the ancient Greek διάγνωσις (diágnōsis), from διαγιγνώσκω (diagignóskō, "to discern"), from διά (diá, "through") + γιγνώσκω (gignóskō, "to know"). We know about a person with the help of information that allows us to see in. When exactly the earliest birth attendants began to notice the connection between the appearance of the rhombus over the female sacrum and the course of childbirth is unknown, but it can be assumed that this connection has been known for a long time. The obstetric textbooks of the 19th century and, probably, of an earlier period described this anatomical phenomenon:

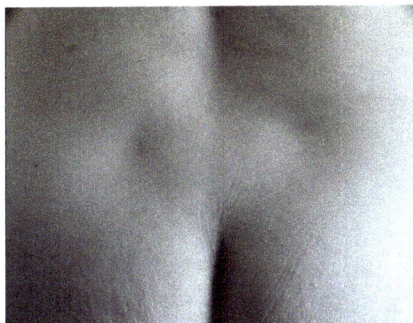

The rhombus of Michaelis, or external appearance of the sacred bone

The lumbosacral rhombus, or rhombus of Michaelis, is a platform on the posterior surface of the sacrum: the upper corner of the rhombus is the recess between the fifth lumbar vertebra and the beginning of the middle sacral crest. Lateral angles correspond to the posterior superior spines of the ilium; lower—the top of the sacrum; on top and outside the rhombus is limited by protrusions of the large spinal muscles, below and outside—by the protrusions of the gluteal muscles. With a normal pelvis, in well-built women, the rhombus is close to a square and is clearly visible when viewed. With the wrong physique and shape of the pelvis, the rhombus is not clearly expressed and its shape changes [26]

This is a fairly clear description of the identification of the rhombus, but remains a mystery: what exactly is the value of knowing the dimensions of the rhombus in a particular woman, besides the most general definition of the possibility of dystocia in childbirth?

The rhombus is valuable in that its shape quite accurately reflects the shape of the pelvic inlet, and also exactly corresponds to the anteroposterior diameter of the inlet and the transverse diameter of the midpelvis. Thus, in many cases, we have the opportunity to determine the type of pelvis, and the morphological type, with only a study of the rhombus.

The examiner finds the transverse points of the rhombus where the dimples (also known as the "dimples of Venus") above the right and left buttocks are visible or felt. It is necessary to compress the thumbs as precisely as possible into these dimples, in order to find the points of indentation on the sacrum. The dimples represent the sacroiliac joints—the points at which the ilia meet the sacrum. A line drawn between the dimples passes over the spinous processes of the second sacral vertebrae. The transverse diameter can be approximated with a fist, which, having measured its width in advance and applied between these points, is a handy measuring device. For a more accurate determination, a measuring tape (in centimeters) may be used. Absence of dimples tell us that the sacrum is flat, which indicates its internal curve is straighter. It is also generally an indication of massive bones.

Massive bones indicate an abundance of minerals, of earth-oriented tendencies: a groundedness, a down-to-earthness. Sometimes this down-to-earthness can become an extreme pragmatism in which the person lacks any strivings toward the higher goals of life. Any of the morphological types can have massive bones but they are more commonly observed in android and android-mix women. Large-boned

---

26   Kaplan A. *Obstetrics.* Moscow, 1954.

women can represent any of the five basic miasms, although they are least commonly observed in tubercular types. Thin bones are associated with poor assimilation of minerals (mostly calcium and phosphorus), and a certain etherealness. They are most commonly observed in gynecoid and anthropoid women. Thin-boned women tend to be associated with the psoric, tubercular, and syphilitic miasms. They tend to have numerous fears and usually express their feelings openly (and sometimes dramatically). Thick-boned women are often extremely sensitive, both emotionally and physically, but tend to hide their feelings.

After giving birth, a woman's rhombus dimples tend to become even more defined, owing to the slight separation and widening that occurs between the bony junctures during birth. The "little cross" expands through the initiation of childbirth.

The transverse diameter of the rhombus is very important for us in that it reflects the transverse diameter of the midpelvis—the so-called "plane of least dimensions." We already know that the minimum size of the transverse diameter of the midpelvis is 10 cm. and so the transverse diameter of the rhombus should also not be less than this for a vaginal birth.

The vertical diameter is also measured from the lower point of the rhombus, which begins approximately where the buttocks crack ends, to the upper edge, which corresponds to the fifth lumbar vertebrae. The anteroposterior diameter (i.e., vertical measurement of the rhombus) is more difficult to determine with the eye, since the lower and upper edges of the rhombus are less clearly visible than the dimples.

During labor a visible change in the rhombus occurs before and during the second stage. It becomes more convex in the middle—the so-called "bulging of the sacrum." This corresponds with the woman seeking positions which allow the sacrum to "lead," to be on top. Therefore, she often chooses to be on hands and knees, or to sit leaning forward. After a woman has given birth at least once, the rhombus changes in proportion to changes in the pelvis; it becomes more visible, and its dimensions increase. The tendency during childbirth for women to keep the sacrum up, to "lead" with the sacrum, is interestingly observed in infants when they are learning to sit, crawl, and stand. They, too, lead with the sacrum: it is the first part that they raise when moving from a sit to a stand, and when they crawl, the sacrum is what they are shifting from side to side (and not just lifting and moving the legs).

The sacrum, in other words, actually houses the center of gravity of the body. When all is well, and it remains the center, the breath is also centered there just above the false pelvis. The centered breath allows for balanced and centered movement, thought, and relationships with the world: together this centeredness allows for second-circle being. Compensatory physical and emotional habits contribute to people shifting the center of gravity to another place. This shift necessarily takes the breath with it.

A rhombus is a mirror of the shape and size of the pelvis when viewed from above. The upper portion corresponds with the posterior sagittal area and the lower part with the anterior side of the pelvis. The shape of the rhombus is the key to the morphological type. As described above, the rhombus is usually close to a square and is clearly visible when viewed. An even square usually indicates a uniformly narrowed gynecoid pelvis (in this case, bone mass should be checked). A small rhombus is associated with contracted pelvis and dystocia in childbirth.[27]

The rhombus of Michaelis, as the external picture of the sacred bone, is clearly visible from birth, both in girls and boys. Any abnormalities in the formation of the pelvic bones can be seen from birth. The midwife checks not only the symmetry of the rhombus in a newborn, but also the symmetry of the skin folds of the thighs (which, if asymmetrical, indicate disbalance in the pelvis) and the folds of fat in the waist area. In women with an adequate pelvis for childbirth, the rhombus is symmetrical. An asymmetric rhombus is an ominous sign and indicates an imbalanced pelvis. During childbirth, massaging the dimples of the rhombus, which is often done intuitively, helps to alleviate discomfort.

---

27   Bansal S, Guleria K, Agarwal N. (2011). "Evaluation of sacral rhomboid dimensions to predict contracted pelvis: a pilot study of Indian primigravidae." *J Obstet Gynaecol India.*;61(5):523-527. doi:10.1007/s13224-011-0078-8

The sacrum is the structure closest to the reproductive organs and the eliminative organs. Elimination of waste from the body can be associated with release of the old, letting go of that which no longer serves us. Elimination and our control of the process implies a relationship with forgiveness of self and others; "letting go." Tightening the pelvic floor muscles closes off the anal sphincter and the urethra, and tightens up the perineal muscles, making a woman's vagina less penetrable. In a woman, the muscles of the pelvic floor, buttocks, and lower abdomen are involved in both elimination (release) and reception. The closing off of our energetic connection to the earth is spiritually and physically unhealthy. A woman who is in a state of being perpetually offended or fearful is not willing or able to receive life support from the earth or inspiration from the world. Her inspiration (literally "breathing in") is stifled and she closes down creatively. The sacred bone area expands with the inspiration of breath to accommodate the abundant love from the created world. Sometimes children are inadvertently trained into closing off the energetic center of the pelvis through rigorous physical training, such as classical ballet.

The work we do with people is relational. Everything is about relationship. Our relationship needs to be authentic, to come from a place of sincerity. The relationship between practitioner and patient needs to be mutual, mindful, present. Being engaged with another implies not only an exchange, but a trinitarian interaction: when everything "works," a third field is created between two people which reflects mutual attentiveness, presence, respect, sincerity, and love. For some, this third element is the Holy Spirit. For this to occur, both parties involved need to be aware of their center of gravity—the sacred bone, holding balance between this world and the next, between the material and the spiritual, between life and death. Our work as practitioners of any kind can encompass, firstly, teaching people about becoming aware of the sacred bone, and then possibly applying our understanding in practice.

Exercises for increasing awareness of and centering in the Sacred Bone

The following exercises benefit any practitioner (and especially birth attendants, but also homeopaths, osteopaths, chiropractors, body workers), as well as those who are interested in finding, developing, or perfecting their true voice in a state of presence (performers, teachers, religious leaders, executive speakers, and all kinds of leaders, as well as people who need healing on any level).

1. Good morning

Stand with the feet just a bit wider than the width of the shoulders. Perform a slight squat while allowing the arms to swing up and to the side, meeting above the head, then on the next squat the arms cross the body and swing down, and circle again as the next squat is performed. The knees should never become locked on the upswing. You can say "Good morning!" in time with the natural breath.

2. Carrying the sun

Stand with the feet at shoulders' width apart and the knees slightly bent. Place all your concentration on your sacrum. Swing your arms up to meet above the head, keeping the elbows bent and forming a circle. With your knees bending as you rotate at the hips, carry the "sun" in the circle of your arms first to one side, and then down to the floor and up to the other side, then carry it in the other direction, always holding your concentration on your sacrum. Do this several times in each direction. At the end, allow the arms to gently come down to your sides, all the while keeping them slightly bent at the elbow and keeping the knees bent as well.

3. Stork walk

Walk around the space, keeping your attention focused on the sacrum, and hiking each hip up very high on each side, thus exaggerating each step. Your legs should be lifted much higher than usual, but the strength of the lift comes from a conscious raising of the hip, rather than a raising of the leg. You can keep your hands on the back of your pelvis in order to help maintain focus. When you walk up stairs at any time, try walking the same way—concentrating on lifting the hips up and keeping the sacrum centered. This exercise really helps with making the sacred bone the center of gravity.

4. Crawling, sitting, and standing up

Get down on hands and knees, and crawl around the floor. Imagine how a toddler crawls. The movement comes from the pelvis; you don't need to consciously lift your legs. From the side, an observer would see your sacrum as "leading," and your legs following as you shift each hip. Move slowly and deliberately, centering all your attention in the sacral area. As a variation, try moving into a sitting position as a toddler does: with your sacrum leading, allow it to fall back from the crawling position onto the floor. Then resume the crawling position in the same way, allowing the sacrum to lead. You can imagine an invisible string pulling your sacrum up from the floor. Try then to stand using the same principle: first you will need to place one foot on the floor while the other leg remains bent in the all-fours position. Allow the sacrum to lead and pull you into a stand. You should feel very much like a small child while doing this (that's how you know you're doing it correctly).

5. Intoning in a deep squat

Standing with your legs widely spaced, go into a deep squat on the floor, leaving your heels flat on the floor if possible. This might require placing your legs even farther apart. Lean on your hands, which are placed on the floor between your legs. This allows the sacrum to rise up a bit and lead. Breathe down low into the floor, and on the exhale, make an "ooo" sound. Send the sound directly down through your pelvis. Experiment with various sounds to see how different sounds influence your awareness of your sacrum.

The sacred bone and positions during labor and birth

The exercises above are very beneficial to do together with a pregnant woman in preparation for labor. During labor it is useful to encourage positions that allow the sacrum to "lead." This implies that the woman leaning slightly forward. Most women intuitively find such positions, if they are allowed to.

Sitting on a birthing ball should be avoided at all costs. Sitting on any object during labor is counterproductive, unless the object has an open center (like a toilet seat or a birthing stool), which puts the weight-bearing on the thighs, and not on the ischia (the "sits bones"). Sitting on the ischia during labor impedes the sacred bone, no matter how soft the seat is (as on a birthing ball), because the coccyx is obligated to curve under. Dealing with contractions while sitting on a birthing ball for long periods of time can have the effect of "jamming" the baby's head into the cavity of the pelvis. The pelvic outlet in such a position is reduced. If the baby is occiput-posterior, the birthing ball can cause the cervix to swell, can lead to overt pressure on the baby's head and spine and potentially lead to hypoxia. It is this author's opinion that they should be completely removed from birthing paraphernalia. A large meta-analysis found that use of the birthing ball does not increase the chance of vaginal delivery.[28]

Even a birthing chair (or a toilet seat) should not be used until the very end of labor, when the baby's head is already visible and is no longer receding between contractions. A birthing chair inhibits blood flow in the mother's thighs and can induce swelling of the vulva. A birthing stool's purpose is only to provide extra support for the woman who might not feel strong enough to birth on hands and knees, or in a supported squat (the latter, too, is best achieved if she is able to maintain a semi-squat, with knees bent about halfway, so that her sacrum in "on top"). A deep squat usually creates undue pressure on the perineum (which should be noted particularly for women of morphological types that have long perineums, i.e., android and anthropoid).

During the descent phase, from full dilatation until the baby's head reaches the pelvic floor, the baby must undergo internal rotation. Internal rotation occurs at the very last, just before the head begins deflexion on its way through the curve of Carus, into the second half of the 90-degree turn, before emerging. This period of descent is the most challenging for the babies, because they undergo an enormous amount of intracranial pressure. God's providence has the process designed such that by the time the cervix is fully dilated and descent begins, the baby falls asleep—owing to the burst of relaxin hormone, which accompanies

---

28   Somayeh Makvandi; Khadigeh Mirzaiinajmabadi; Najmeh Tehranian; Masoumeh Mirteimouri; Ramin Sadeghi. (2019). "The impact of birth ball exercises on mode of delivery and length of labor: A systematic review and meta-analysis". *Journal of Midwifery and Reproductive Health*, 7, 3, 1718-1727. doi: 10.22038/jmrh.2019.33781.1367

the high oxytocin level, that takes place at this time. The baby's sleep is indicated by lack of movement. If the baby exhibits dramatic movement after 8 cm dilatation, it is a sign that the position is likely occiput-posterior and the contractions have become weaker (less oxytocin is being released, as well as less relaxin). The occiput-posterior baby will eventually fall asleep, but only if contractions resume their strength and relaxin is once again stimulated. This increase in strength is what is needed, too, for the head to reach the pelvic floor, where it will finally undergo internal rotation in all but 5% of persistent-posterior positions.[29] In the case of a posterior baby, this entails, usually, a long-arc rotation of 135° into the occiput-anterior position.

The side-lying position during labor is useful when the woman is tired or when the baby is occiput-posterior. Side-lying with the upper leg bent at the hip and flexed as high as possible upward, and allowed to rest on a large pillow, gives the sacrum maximum space. Most women in this position will begin to spontaneously turn over to hands and knees with the increase in contraction strength.

Being aware of the role of the sacred bone in labor (and otherwise) as the center of gravity and the energetic center of the physical body, is essential in therapeutic work. The rhombus provides the specifics about this particular sacred bone and this particular morphology. Adjusting one's focus and increasing attention to this center is usually all that is needed for major healing change to occur. The heretofore application of reductionistic thought in medicine, in midwifery and even—unfortunate as it is—in all manner of therapeutic work, has led to viewing every aspect of life, every part of the human body, every stage in labor, or every minute section of human physiology or psyche, as separate. This way of interpreting every process and every part as merely "process" or "part" is blind to any whole, to any totality. Even the so-called holistic therapies

---

29   Chloé Dole, Jean Patrick Metz, Justine Formet, Didier Riethmuller, Rajeev Ramanah, Nicolas Mottet. (2021). "Intra pelvic spontaneous rotation of persistent occiput posterior position in case of operative vaginal delivery with spatulas." *Journal of Gynecology Obstetrics and Human Reproduction*, Volume 50, Issue 2.

are so only in name, insofar as they do not regard a hierarchy of any level. There is no acknowledgment of that which holds it all together. Attention to (and even acknowledgment of) the force that organizes the hierarchy of being, on every level, is missing. It is not seen. Therefore, we witness no unifying cosmology about human existence and, consequently, about health and disease and healing. Interpretations are all local and limited. Where there is no overarching understanding, all understandings are just well-defended personal opinions, one-sided and not far-seeing. We can't see, for the most part, love—that is, God— as the energy attracting all things to each other and holding all things together. This God—as love— permeates every piece of our being and those pieces are incarnated love, love manifested, in specific forms, specific morphological designs. The form reflects the meaning. It's all there, plain as day.

This knowledge was innate for our forebears. The price of the age of reason was a suppression of intuitive knowledge. Now reason has all but overtaken us. We have come full circle, and now the once-intuitive needs to be made conscious.

CHAPTER FIVE.

What We Are Observing

The obstetricians who first recorded information about pelvimetry made note that certain pelvic types are more prevalent among certain ethnic groups around the world. The gynecoid type is the most prevalent everywhere. The anthropoid type is more common among African peoples. The platypelloid type is most commonly found among Asian ethnic groups. Android women are more common in northern and southern Europe.

Early obstetricians used their classification system to make prognoses about birth, especially for primiparous women. Before the safety of operative delivery, doctors and midwives were concerned with one question above all others: can this baby be born through this pelvis and will the mother survive? In borderline situations, the question became: can this baby be born by forceps through this pelvis? The hope of midwives has always been that a healthy baby will be born to a healthy mother, but how quickly we forget that not so long ago, birth attendants had the main goal of ensuring that the mother, at least, would survive. Safe operative delivery changed everything; practitioners' need for rigorous clinical prognostic abilities fell by the wayside. But it also changed evolution: *morphologically nonadaptive pelvic traits would now be passed down to children together with the myriad of miasmatic and constitutional traits associated with them.* This is an important point often overlooked in the natural-birth and holistic-health sphere. As many as five generations of women have now birthed by cesarean section and five generations of children have changed the genetic and morphological mix of humankind.

The prognosis of a particular woman's labor depends, among other things, on the type and shape of the pelvis. These observations undoubtedly provided an enormous contribution to the art of midwifery. Yet this realm of science—pelvimetry—remains to this day specialized and narrow; it addresses the specific physical form of the pelvis, without taking into account the ways in which the pelvis relates to other characteristic elements of the person, or the person as a totality.

Neither modern midwifery, its claims to holistic practice notwithstanding, nor obstetrics offers an all-encompassing model for classification and a simple, effective system for making a prognosis about the course of labor in nulliparous women. The "parts" are still considered in exclusion of one another. If the physical classification was paramount just over 100 years ago, it gave way to a no less lopsided bias for the psychological-spiritual by the end of the 20th century, which persists to this day. If the paucity of life-saving medical technology gave rise, then, to a concentration on the physical process, the overuse of medical technology, now, has given rise to a disregard for the physical (and among midwives an over-emphasis on the psychological). Both extremes are inaccurate. Neither approach is holistic. The *individual* is invisible. Even homeopathy, with its all-encompassing holistic view of the person, lacks knowledge about a total morphology of the person (although some homeopaths apply "facial analysis" or body-type models). This results in a generalized, non-individualistic approach to prevention, treatment, and analysis, and a less-than-complete understanding about what we encounter in practice. Pelvimetry, as a system of classification, was relatively recently discovered—as it happens, on the eve of the paradigm shift in scientific and medical consciousness toward materialism and reductionism. It never had the chance to come to ripeness. Twenty-first-century consciousness hypothetically offers fertile ground to incorporate much of what has been gleaned from discrete medical specialties. The beauty of morphology lies in its universal applicability for all healing/therapeutic modalities.

Ancient Greek medicine had an appreciation for and knowledge of typology: the physical constitution and its various parts were classified and correlated with the four temperaments, the four humors, the four elements, the four faculties, the vital principles, the four administering virtues, and the organs and parts. Greek medicine was first codified and systematized by the Greek philosopher-physician Hippocrates in the 4th century BCE. and subsequently developed and expanded by other physicians, most notably Galen, Dioscorides, and Avicenna. Hippocrates was known to have said, "Through the like, disease is produced and through the application of the like, it is cured."

Morphological types, homeopathic constitutions and miasms, and circles of energy

A *symptom*, in homeopathic understanding, is an inherent expression, a characteristic, a trait, an attribute. Symptoms are not consciously chosen. They merely individualize a person. For example, symptoms include things like: all the details of one's physical appearance; the kind of weather one prefers, and the season; the time of day one feels best or worst; food preferences and aversions; sleep habits; menstrual regularity; all emotional and mental expressions and reactions; digestive problems and tendencies; degree of perspiration; sexual desire; physical illnesses; and so on.

People place value markers on their own and others' symptoms, rather than being honest:

"What foods do you like most?"

"Well, I avoid meat, since it's bad for you, you know it causes cancer and heart disease, and of course I stay away from sugar because it destroys the blood vessels."

"But what do you *like*?"

"What do I like? I like all kinds of Middle Eastern sweets like loukoum and baklava, but don't eat them!"

This example reveals two symptoms: a desire for sweets, and also a fixed understanding about health (which if probed further might uncover an outright anxiety about health, or a desire to "do the correct thing," or a desire to appear educated, and so on). The explaining away, or rationalization of a symptom, is what homeopaths might call a *comfort story*. Comfort stories are people's way of more rationally (or so it seems) understanding why things are as they are. They include physical ailments as well. Many comfort stories are culturally based. In Russia, for example, there is an inordinate emphasis on the danger of drafts, especially cross-winds, and they take the blame for every possible symptom. Mediterranean cultures have the "evil eye" to explain why bad things happen. Modern comfort stories, created by modern medicine and subsequently becoming oral tradition in our era, include blaming micro-organisms for our ills. "I was sitting in a crowded bus and I think there were all kinds of viruses around and I caught one." The point is not that these stories don't contain an element of truth, but that they omit the whole picture. The whole picture always includes one's miasmatic heritage which relates to a great degree to one's susceptibility. Symptoms are unfolding from within, not imposed on us from without. We are acorns becoming oaks, not empty vessels being filled whichever way the wind blows.

Symptoms show the vital force in action. The vital force elicits symptoms—whatever their nature may be—always "doing what it can with what it's got," with the purpose of achieving balance. A symptom is not good or bad, it just *is*. Homeopaths accept them phenomenologically. This approach trains us to practice presence and unconditional love. We begin by observing, without judgment, classification, or a knee-jerk reaction to make the symptom go away.

A *constitution* is an array of symptoms making up a totality that expresses the essence of a person at the given time. Constitutions are fewer in number than symptoms, being higher in the hierarchy of life, and therefore many people share a specific constitution at a given time in their life. For example, a lemon, a grapefruit, and a lime all share many symptoms, and one could say they all have the citrus constitution. Symptoms, therefore, are always nearly endless in number, while constitutions are more limited in their potential expressions. A constitution is always a *totality*: a whole that is greater than the sum of its parts (= symptoms). All beings on earth are totalities. We recognize a person as a totality, and never as merely a group of characteristics. Only totalities can have relationships with one another. Their relationship is characterized by their degree of similarity *as totalities*. People use the phrases "I can really relate to that person," and "I really identify with her." These are expressions of sensing similarity with another. The similarity we find in our friends, or in books, or films, or experiences—the feeling that someone or something "strikes a chord"—is indeed the experience of *resonance* of two vibrational fields. This resonance is itself homeopathic healing: the resonance can become a "resounding" resonance, intensifying the particular vibrational expression and to a certain extent bringing it to fruition. All of life is a series of our striving toward finding resonance with the world around us, finding "chords" that heal our implicate intent!

All beings in the hierarchy of creation, since they are connected in an overarching macrocosm held together by God, have *some* degree of similarity. What we can say is that a totality can't be *opposite* to another totality. John can never be the "opposite" of Jane. Their symptoms might be completely different, when taken apart, but as complex wholes they cannot be true opposites. Any relationship between people is characterized merely by the *degree* of similarity. The symptom-totality is intensified by the *action* of the homeopathic substance (or by the relationship with the Other), according to the degree of similarity between the two, calling into effect Newton's third law and bringing about an equal and opposite *reaction*, through which the symptoms (partially or completely) resolve.

In midwifery practice, a very common complication among primiparous women is labor dystocia (weak contractions). It is so frequent in fact that it is considered normal for first-time mothers. Weakness can occur in first-stage labor (and is known as primary labor dystocia) or in second-stage labor (and is known as secondary labor dystocia). The allopathic treatment (which is also used by most midwives without their being aware of its possible ramifications) is to apply the principle of opposites: a substance or a recommendation is given that strengthens contractions. In a hospital setting this is obviously synthetic and chemical in nature (intravenous synthetic oxytocin or prostaglandins). A homeopathic approach would include recommendations and substances that intensify the weakness, thus applying the law of similars: having the woman rest, do all she can to wait, sleep, and "forget" about labor; and of course the ingestion of a homeopathic medicine which in material doses causes weak labor contractions (together with her other symptoms at this time). The law of similars encourages us as midwives to "hold back" on stimulating contractions as much as possible. We have the woman lie on her side, turn off the lights, and leave her alone for a period of time, and this has the effect of "winding up the spring" of the symptoms of weak contractions, intensifying them, until her body has reached its fulfillment of this symptom (i.e., latent intent), and then labor intensifies. The same principle applies to relationships: "absence makes the heart grow fonder," "familiarity breeds contempt." A relationship that has been very intimate in every sphere very quickly more easily plays itself out—two people "heal" each other's symptoms intensely, the symptom-picture of each subsequently changes, and the degree of similarity is less ("we outgrew each other"). In this regard, what most people consider love is really attraction rooted in the satisfaction of finding one's homeopathic remedy in the form of another person.

A *miasm*, as opposed to a *constitution*, is a more general grouping of many different constitutions into one of several general categories. According to the homeopathic theory of miasms, each person is born with a certain spectrum of predispositions, or adaptive mechanisms, which during life are manifested depending on external and internal factors. Homeopaths classify these predispositions into several general groups. The founder of homeopathy, Samuel Hahnemann, elucidated through his practice and observation three main miasmatic groups. The word miasm comes from the Greek and means "pollution, stain." Hahnemann believed that the miasms leave a sort of stain on the constitution of a person, thereby determining the specific ways in which the person will respond to the environment. Behind all of the chronic diseases are miasms, which are either inherited or acquired in life.

Miasms create a barrier to the vital force that prevent it from adequately achieving equilibrium. Miasms are wider than what we know as "genetic predispositions," since they encompass physical, emotional, and mental tendencies. They are the cause of chronic illness. There is no person born without a dominant miasm, and many people's leading miasm changes in the course of their lifetime. Classical homeopathic treatment aims to mitigate congenital miasms. While there is no such thing as a person with no illness, homeopathic treatment helps to bring chronic tendencies to fruition, thereby reducing the likelihood of their being expressed as overt pathology.

It is absolutely essential to grasp the concept put forth by homeopathy that the vital force, no matter what it does and no matter which symptoms or illnesses it manifests, always and everywhere seeks balance for the person. The vital force cannot therefore be "weak," "faulty," or "mistaken." Whatever we see in the form of symptoms, then, is the vital force's attempt at bringing about well-being. This is nearly impossible to integrate as a concept, since we have been indoctrinated to seek "causes" of our misery (which, we were taught, is what illness is—misery). This homeopathic rock is the basis on which all of the art stands. When we regard the vital force as only "correct," we change our attitudes about illness, and about patients. The fact that sometimes symptoms lead to death is not because the vital force is mistaken, but because it does what it can with what it has, and all people are fallible, mortal, and flawed.

More than 200 years after Hahnemann, the miasms can be grouped into five major types. Each miasm is itself a totality, behind each of which stands a unifying "theme" or motivating drive or goal. Once again, these drives or goals are specific forms of self-actualization (bringing the symptom-totality to fruition, thus closer to one's divine image) for each individual. They are not chosen consciously. *They go beyond psychological wounds and subconscious choices.* On the contrary: the way one expresses his or her woundedness (or one might say: the wounds we attract to ourselves) is determined by our dominant miasm. Miasms represent collective patterns of implicate intent, necessary for the person's healing (actualization of the soul, theosis, growing toward the divine image in which one was created).

Miasms (and on the more individual level constitutions and symptoms) can be considered the individual path on which one is journeying (the *tropos*) or fate. Three somewhat distinct forces shape the lives of people in Homer's *Odyssey*: fate, intervention from the gods, and the actions of the people themselves. For homeopathy, each person is born with a dominant miasm (fate) or spectrum of potential pathology, world view, and desires. In *The Odyssey*, though the gods seem all-powerful, the goddess Athena herself admits: "The great leveler, Death: not even the gods can defend a man, not even one they love, that day when fate takes hold and lays him out at last." The inherited dominant miasm determines the character of the road one will be on, but free will, the nature of the journey as one's fate unfolds—whether it will be difficult or easy, full of shame or glory—depends on God's grace (God's will) and human will. The Beatitudes of Jesus Christ are called in Russian заповеди блаженства—"commandments of grace", emphasizing not only their nature as gift from God but also as commandments, the fulfillment of which assists the person in living an honorable, grace-filled life, miasm notwithstanding!

Miasms are manifest in the person at conception and may be considered inherited tendencies. According to homeopathic philosophy these tendencies are not understood in quite the same way as they are by genetics and current science. They reflect *unfulfilled intent*, or symptom-pictures that did not come to fruition, were not resolved, in the previous generations. One might regard these tendencies as the "sins of the fathers" that were never quite rooted out. The vital force works across generations to bring to fulfillment particular tendencies, just as it works within an individual toward the same end, and symptoms that are suppressed, or not resolved, lead to the vital force eventually finding a deeper level in the organism for expression. Sometimes this deeper level means manifesting the tendency in the offspring. In this respect, the appearance of a particular miasmatic expression—according to homeopathic theory—is not just the result of random gene combinations, but is the natural result of suppression. Patterns we observe in our patients are not random but expected, even predictable. This knowledge influences our attitude toward symptoms and illness and helps us to regard them as the *means to a potentially glorious end*, rather than a curse.

Each miasm was discovered as the chronic expression of an acute illness. Hahnemann originally thought that the origin of psora is the Sarcoptes scabiei mite, which produces the scabies illness. Scabies, he believed, was a disease capable of becoming chronic in the individual and persisting throughout a person's lifetime, showing its influence in a specific group of symptoms. The sycotic miasm is the chronic form of gonorrhea, with which the individual or his relatives suffered at some point in time and which was suppressed, thus passing it on as a chronic taint to successive generations. The same is true of the syphilitic miasm: the chronic disease tendencies created by syphilis, either in the individual or in the family line, are easily identified and difficult to root out. The **tubercular** miasm is a chronic trend that starts with a parent or grandparent having suffered with tuberculosis. The **cancer** miasm is well known for being passed down in families, although what homeopaths understand as the cancer miasm does not always express itself in actual oncological disease, just as the acute diseases associated with the other miasms are not required for the miasmatic diagnosis and don't guarantee that the person will come down with that illness.

Knowledge about miasms changes the way one sees oneself and others. Within each miasm are detailed, specific features that reach far past disease history. Sometimes it is enough to know what an ancestor did for a living, where they chose to live, what kind of hobbies and interests they had, and what kind of stories are associated with them to identify the dominant miasm. Having knowledge about the chronic illnesses of our ancestors also helps, but not all diseases are associated solely with one miasm. Miasms are, once again, *totalities*. A totality is always greater than the sum of its parts. We might examine a family, for example, or the members of a dance club, or a class of adult students all taking the same course—and determine the leading element that unites all of them. We identify their similarities, and also make note of what distinguishes one from another. Within one group we would probably find more similarities than differences.

	Psoric	Sycotic	Syphilitic	Tubercular	Cancer
Main theme	Survival	Reproduction	Disconnection	Search	Immortality
Period of life exemplified	Infancy and childhood	Young adult-hood	Old age	Generally teen years but can be lifelong	Lifelong
Personality tendencies	Dependent, fearful, reliable	Values outer appearances, seeks growth	Dependent/independent, self-destructive	Seeks change, spiritual joy, creative, home-sick	Nonacceptance of self, rebels against self, strives to be perfect
Statement	"I'm afraid"	"How do I look?"	"I'll do it myself"	"Seek and you shall find"	"I must do it perfectly"
Body build	Average	Tends to gain weight	Heavy-set or very lean	Average-lean	Average

Over the years since Hahnemann, several homeopaths have suggested a wider variety of miasms, some having suggested as many as 14 or more. If we apply the working definition of a miasm as a taint on the constitution, a block to the action of vital force which prevents it from reaching the fruition of its strivings, then miasm can be seen as anything that does just that. Some homeopaths have observed that certain other diseases leave such a long-term "taint" and barrier to cure, that they must be classified as miasmatic illnesses, and the chronic symptom picture thereafter as a miasmatic picture. Such barriers can be acquired during one's lifetime; for example, after taking certain medications or vaccines, some people's vital force cannot overcome the barrier thus induced—this could be termed an acquired medicinal miasm. Some people's vital force cannot recover after a serious illness (Covid-19, meningitis, Lyme disease, for example), or following an emotional upheaval (fright, trauma, grief); these would also be classified as acquired miasms, blocks that need to be homeopathically treated and cured before the vital force can move on. Of the chronic, inherited miasms, however, most homeopaths of our time agree that there are five indisputable ones which can be observed in practice over and over again.

Caldwell and Moloy's classification of the pelvic types persists to this day, but the extensive contributions from classical midwifery and homeopathy can now be united in a new, more all-encompassing model. What was previously limited to knowledge about the pelvis and its influence on the course of labor and birth can now be expanded to all facets of a woman's being. Having come so far from the reductionist age in medicine and science, now we ask questions about interrelatedness within the person and between people, between groups of people and nations, between humankind as a whole and God. Here we ask: what are the relationships between pelvic type, overall morphological type, constitution, and miasm? We can take it even farther: knowledge about morphology, constitution, and miasms can be extended to areas outside childbirth and women. The discrete mode of understanding the human being has given way to holism, just as human experience also is changing from a linear cause-and-effect mentality toward the "field" mentality of quantum physics.

As discussed earlier, holistic understanding presupposes a certain *entelechy* at work in every person: each person is an ever-becoming soul, undergoing a dynamic process of incarnation with his or her specific "form" or "idea" that is continuously being realized, and also awaits ultimate realization—like the towering oak tree in the tiny acorn. The "form" awaiting expression represents the perfect image of the person, God's "idea" that was the prototype for the person's creation. The prototype being of course the God-man Jesus Christ, the original *Logos* (word) after whose image we are fashioned. All people, in turn, contain within themselves what St. Maximus the Confessor called their own *logos*.[30]

---

30   Logos, (Greek: "word," "reason," or "plan") plural logoi, in ancient Greek philosophy and early Christian theology, the divine reason implicit in the cosmos, ordering it and giving it form and meaning.

The *logoi of creation* reflect the divine image of all beings that make up the cosmos, as they each have their origin in God and bear similarity to Him. "In the beginning was the Word, and the word was with God, and the word was God" (John 1:1). Each person was created by a benevolent and loving God in His own image. While the divine image (*logos*) is given from our creation, the divine likeness (*tropos*) is something we must strive toward achieving. The *tropos* leads to the *logos*.

Homeopathic philosophy corroborates this idea. In homeopathy we "see" the symptom-picture, the *tropos* of the person, and it is the *tropos* that we aim to facilitate, while all the time striving to see the divine *logos* of the person behind the symptoms. Since every person is created in God's image, each also possesses divine qualities—however, the sinful (mortal) state of humankind prevents us from a pure expression of these qualities. Instead we display symptoms—which can be viewed as nothing more than *altered divine qualities* manifested by the vital force in an attempt to achieve equilibrium and ultimately a return to God.

The acknowledgment of the divine origin of every person, together with each one's *implicate intent* (i.e., divine image striving toward realization) is extremely important in the healing arts. It puts the practitioner on the proverbial train platform, imagining in detail what the journey will look like, and this is in direct opposition to our habitual cause-and-effect reasoning which searches for needles in haystacks as "causes" of a disease process we currently observe. We begin to regard what we currently observe as the explicate expression of a latent intent that had been in the person all along—like the characteristic shape of the leaves of an oak tree. We begin to see where they are going and then may ask ourselves how we are facilitating their becoming.

When health practitioners acknowledge implicate intent, they are admitting to several things:

1. That each person has a specific and relatively predefined mode of eventual actualization (within general limitations);

2. That, since one person's trouble areas are specific, there is very little room for random "accidents";

3. That a healthy, personal actualization of implicate intent constitutes a fulfilled life; and therefore

4. That random suppression of this actualization (through suppression of symptoms) is detrimental to the soul.

For midwifery, the law of suppression reveals the potential harm of procedures such as anesthetised childbirth, abortion, cesarean section, cervical dilatation and curettage, across-the-board hormonal "therapy," suppression of menopause, unnecessary hysterectomy, and on and on; and why these suppressive actions have profound consequences for a woman not only at the level of the body, but at the level of the psyche. While suppression is not always avoidable (and indeed implies free will and choice), nevertheless it is essential to acknowledge its effects, and to courageously make prognoses, as healthcare providers, which include likely reactions to those suppressions. Beyond that there is also the question of informed consent.

For example: a woman suffers from chronic yeast infections after having taken antibiotics several times over the course of a few years for cystitis. Along with yeast infections she started suffering from mood swings. Her gynecologist prescribed anti-yeast medications which suppress the symptoms temporarily, only to have them return again and again. In addition, while using the anti-yeast drugs, her psychological state deteriorates even more, her libido has dwindled down to nothing, and she now suffers from new physical symptoms (any number of possibilities could be manifested). Her doctors regard her as having x-disease at any given time, not recognizing the relationship with her other symptoms. Her current state is the expression of a chronology of events, with which her vital force has been dealing in the most optimal (and only possible) way. A series of suppressed symptoms led to her current state. Had she treated her original condition homeopathically, it would have been brought to fruition, realized, and it would have been over and done with. Now, what we witness is not in fact what we think it is, but rather a suppressed cystitis. With homeopathic treatment, the symptoms of cystitis will return very briefly, at which time they can be healed properly—through the law of similars. That is, the cure for her yeast infections (and the mood swings that attended them) is her cystitis!

The acknowledgment that what we are observing in a person is the *manifestation of a necessity* helps us to see patterns more clearly, to understand the true etiology of a problem. It means that every diagnosis with which a patient comes to us is under scrutiny. It alters our entire manner of diagnosis and prognosis. Therefore, it alters our approach to cure. When, for example, a woman tells the story of her previous pregnancy and birth, during which she carried the baby to 42 weeks and 2 days gestation and then her labor began with spontaneous rupture of membranes and an abnormally lengthy preliminary phase—we infer that she is likely of android morphology, probably sycotic miasm, implying a likely yeast infection (or other infection of the urogenital system) with a posterior baby, which is the "diagnosis" we would have given at the onset of labor. At the hospital she would have been diagnosed simply with postdates pregnancy and premature rupture of the membranes. The latter diagnosis is descriptive, but not all-encompassing. She will probably not be informed that her baby is posterior (much less why), which explains her long and painful labor. Because her caregivers were not paying any attention to her morphology, they had not made a prognosis about what was likely to happen and therefore couldn't have prepared the woman, either—and wouldn't have given any recommendations to avoid complications. In homeopathy practice such stories abound. The parent of a child needing homeopathic care tells us in detail about "what happened."

What we can *do* with what we are *observing* is key; after all, having the most complete possible understanding of the *nature of a condition* gives us the possibility of improving that condition. People are not blank slates. Every individual processes experience, and reacts to the environment, in his or her own specific way in accordance with the *tropos* of an individual soul.

CHAPTER SIX.

Gynecoid Morphology

The gynecoid morphology is considered to be the most widespread among women. It is the "common denominator" of female morphology. It is also considered the ideal of female beauty: the Venus de Milo (Aphrodite) statues and images provide typical examples of gynecoid morphology. Notably, Venus' figure does not necessarily reflect the current concept of ideal feminine beauty but rather echoes an ideal from the past. She is not at all the thin, nearly anorexic woman of modern fashion journals, but rather carries noticeable fat in places that accentuate her curves. Her bust size is modest yet proportional, and her hips are clearly the widest part of her figure. In general, she exhibits a wonderful gentleness and grace of lines. Most women exhibit a mixed morphological picture which includes at least some gynecoid elements.

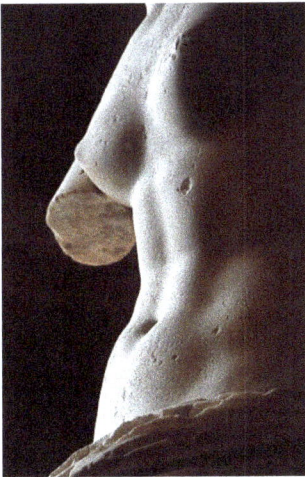

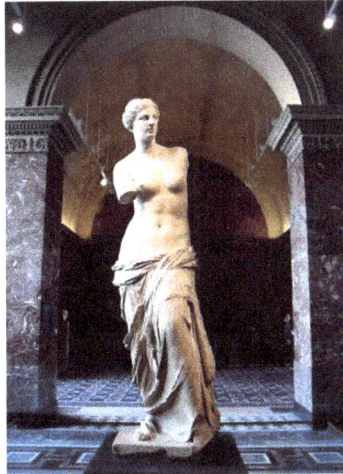

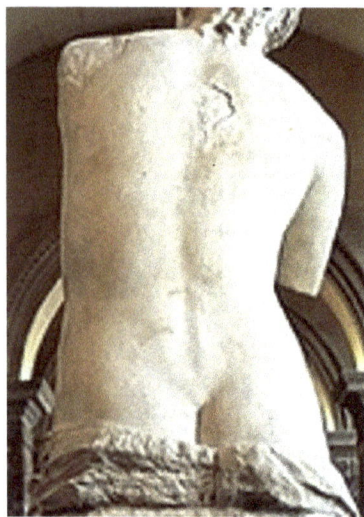

The rhombus of the Venus de Milo is clearly not anatomically correct. In place of a cross shape it exhibits only the "v" above the buttocks and a low-set vertebral column.

Facial features of the gynecoid woman are neither large nor small, are light and well-formed—the chin is not small and not protruding. The shoulders are neither wide nor narrow, sloping from the neck downward, tilted down when viewed from the side. They are narrower than her hips. The average length of her forearm from the elbow to the tip of the middle finger is exactly the same as described in the Bible: one *elbow* (an ancient linear measure of length equal to 42–45 cm, i.e., the length from the elbow to the tip of the longest finger). The fingers are relatively long and thin. She has light and not wide palms. Her "bucket-carrying capacity"[31] is quite adequate—that is, the elbows do not touch the waist when walking.

The hips of a gynecoid woman are wider than her shoulders. The legs taper symmetrically from the hips to the feet, but the inner sides of the thighs and knees do not meet when she is standing with her ankles touching—a likely sign of a sufficient or wide transverse diameter of the cavity and pelvic outlet.

Gynecoid women have natural endurance and stamina, allowing them to easily endure pregnancy and childbirth. Chloasma (hyperpigmentation of the skin of the face in the form of yellowish-brown spots) and the *linea nigra* (the hyper-pigmented line from the navel to the pubis

---

31   "Bucket-carrying capacity" is a concept described by some obstetricians of the early 20th century in the West and it refers to the level of the waist, on the one hand, in combination with the laxity of the ligaments, on the other. Hyperlaxity of ligaments causes the arm to slightly turn inside-out at the elbow when straightened (as in when carrying buckets of water), which causes the elbows to scrape against the waist. Normal laxity does not have such an effect.

Gynecoid Morphology

of a woman in the second half of pregnancy) are often pronounced.[32] This hyperpigmented line can be present not only in pregnant women (although it is far more often observed in these) but also in men and adolescents, and its presence is correlated with higher levels of sex hormones. Hyperpigmentation is a sign of an almost exclusively gynecoid woman, and therefore gives a reliable prognosis for normal childbirth, since a gynecoid woman has a roomy pelvis and labor activity, as a rule, is strong. The teeth of such a woman are usually relatively straight, and the arch of the teeth is semi-circular. The size of the shoe is average for the height. Her height is usually average for her nationality, being neither excessively short nor tall of stature. Her weight, too, tends to be average. She is not thin and not fat. She tends to carry most of her weight in the buttocks and thighs and will gain weight there first.

Her rhombus of Michaelis is always clearly visible and has a classic shape: that of a cross, with the top half of the vertical line just slightly shorter than the lower. Controversial as it is to state, the Venus de Milo when viewed from behind surprisingly does not exhibit a clearly defined rhombus, and the shape of the sacrum is generally not anatomically correct, the lumbar vertebrae clearly beginning far too low. There seems to be no recognition of this fact in the literature, although mention has been made that the shape of the Venus' spine might suggest scoliosis, that her legs are different lengths, and that her face has asymmetrical features.[33]

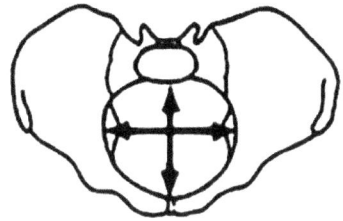

The gynecoid pelvis.

The pelvic brim is rounded at the front, side, and back. The transverse diameter of the pelvic brim is slightly larger than the anteroposte-

32   George, A. O., Shittu, O. B., Enwerem, E., Wachtel, M., & Kuti, O. (2005). "The incidence of lower mid-trunk hyperpigmentation (linea nigra) is affected by sex hormone levels." *Journal of the National Medical Association*, 97(5), 685–688.

33   Andrew, K., Iwanaga, J., Loukas, M., Chapman, J., Oskouian, R. J., & Tubbs, R. S. (2018). "Does the Venus de Milo have a Spinal Deformity?" *Cureus, 10*(8), e3219. https://doi.org/10.7759/cureus.3219

rior diameter of the brim. The posterior sagittal diameter is only slightly shorter than the anterior sagittal diameter of the brim. The sacrum is parallel to the symphysis. The sciatic notch is well rounded, allowing 2.5–3 finger-breadths between the sciatic spine and the sacrum. The walls of the pelvis are straight in relation to each other. The ischial spines are dull, neither sharp not encroaching. The pubic arch is adequate—approximately 90°, no more, no less.

Gynecoid morphology and the psoric miasm

Gynecoid morphology, as the most common type, is most often observed paired with the psoric miasm. A psoric woman is focused on survival and therefore on security and safety. Psoric women have numerous fears, as they feel a subconscious threat to their existence. They need and appreciate the support of others and therefore a pregnant gynecoid-psoric type will definitely expect her partner to be present at the birth. She will insist they attend prenatal classes together. In general, gynecoid-psoric types are affectionate, loving, open, trusting. They are comfortable in second-circle relationships and easily cultivate presence. If they have experienced emotional abuse, rejection, or grief, however, they tend to revert to a first-circle, inward-directed stance and sometimes it is very challenging to win their trust again.

This morphological type tends to give birth around her estimated due date or slightly after, and rarely prematurely. They don't tend to hurry in anything they do, and birth is no exception. Her baby usually settles into the pelvis in the LOA (left occipital anterior) or ROA (right occipital anterior) position. Her ample pelvis allows the baby to drop well ahead of labor (in a primiparous woman), and her cervix begins shortening and effacing in the expected time. Since her baby is almost always anterior, and therefore the head exerts equal pressure on the cervix and on the bony pelvis, she is not likely to have premature rupture of the membranes, unless she has a chronic vaginal infection (candida, for example), which would influence the integrity of the amniotic membranes. The gynecoid woman has a short-to-average length perineum and an average muscle mass, both of which predispose her to giving birth without lacerations. Sometimes her muscles seem flaccid or flabby since the psoric gynecoid woman is not a huge fan of physical exercise. She will exercise for the sake of her health, or from the motivation of wanting to do the right thing, but she is rarely a sports fanatic.

This type of woman can easily "rest on her laurels" once she feels secure in her relationship with her significant other. She does not demand too much of her partner, other than receiving attention and affection, which are primary. If her partner is a cold, reserved type, she might eventually become anxious and even suspicious about her status, since safety and security for her are paramount. This motivation can lead to codependence or a severe neediness, not always expressed in the most healthful manner. In this regard she can also become too dependent on the midwife or other caregiver, especially if she does not feel support from her partner. Such neediness might be expressed as manipulation. It can be a challenge for the caregiver to insist that such a woman take responsibility for herself and her life process, while at the same time remaining patient and loving. This neediness often shows up during labor, especially in primiparous women.

A nulliparous gynecoid woman tends to labor as in the textbooks, with labor lasting 8–18 hours including the preliminary phase. The primiparous gynecoid woman may display a hint of weak labor activity, but usually the situation does not reach the need for augmentation. Such a woman needs a certain degree of reassurance, physical contact, and the presence of loved ones, and which soothe and reassure her. She is beneficially influenced by praise, as she tends to have a bit of insecurity about her abilities. The gynecoid woman is trusting and desires to do whatever is asked of her, as security and safety have an important place in her life. She is ready to do whatever the midwife says. She shows her feelings quite openly. In the transitional phase of childbirth, she usually loses her self-confidence, begins to doubt her ability to give birth, becomes quite weepy and emotional, and expresses sensitivity to pain. If she is scolded or criticized, she is quite easily offended and withdraws into her shell. During labor with a primiparous gynecoid woman this could result in prolonged labor, since the release of cortisol accompanies tension and fear, inhibiting oxytocin release and weakening contractions.

Such women don't tend to be dominant in a relationship. They are considerate and respectful partners and, unless in a decompensated state, attract to themselves equally considerate and respectful people. When in a weakened mental state, such women may attract partners who are domineering, often even emotionally abusive, since they are easily taken advantage of and cannot always defend themselves. She is a persistent learner, does not give up easily, and once she has mastered a task, she copes with it well. They are "trudgers" and will persist with a tedious task faithfully.

Such a woman responds beautifully to the presence of a supportive partner during childbirth, and is also quite comfortable if the husband is the leader in the family. His confidence is very important to her. If he is unsure of himself, confused by all sorts of fears, she will be lost and become indecisive and irritable. In this case, she derives support from the confident leadership of the midwife or another birth partner. When in an uncompensated state, the gynecoid-psoric woman can become excessively needy and dependent, or self-pitying. While it is tempting for her loved ones and for her birth team to give in to her need for constant reassurance, she is far better assisted in her personal growth if she is allowed to experience her own strength. This implies letting her experience the difficulties of giving birth without taking the experience away from her. A woman giving birth in the hospital, for example, might begin to beg for epidural anesthesia; while her dramatic behavior would encourage her birth attendants to concede, their gentle but firm refusal goes a long way toward the woman's ultimate actualization. Anesthesia denies the woman of the full actualization of the childbirth experience. Unless it is medically indicated, it has the effect of undermining a woman's self-confidence, reinforcing her emotional and physical dependence, and suppressing her complete and genuine expression. Natural childbirth gives her opportunity to discover for herself not only what she is capable of emotionally, but discloses the wondrous abilities of her body and this absolutely changes the way she relates to herself. She is ultimately challenged with remaining present with herself and her body.

She is given room to find her true and natural voice. The powerful vocal expression that manifests when the throat and birth canal find connection in the last stage of birth cannot be replaced by any other human life experience. When birth attendants know this, and acknowledge the vital role of natural childbirth for the woman's actualization, they then understand the severe deleterious consequences of anesthetised labor. A gynecoid-psoric woman does not always choose a home birth during her first pregnancy. She looks to her support team for direction. For the

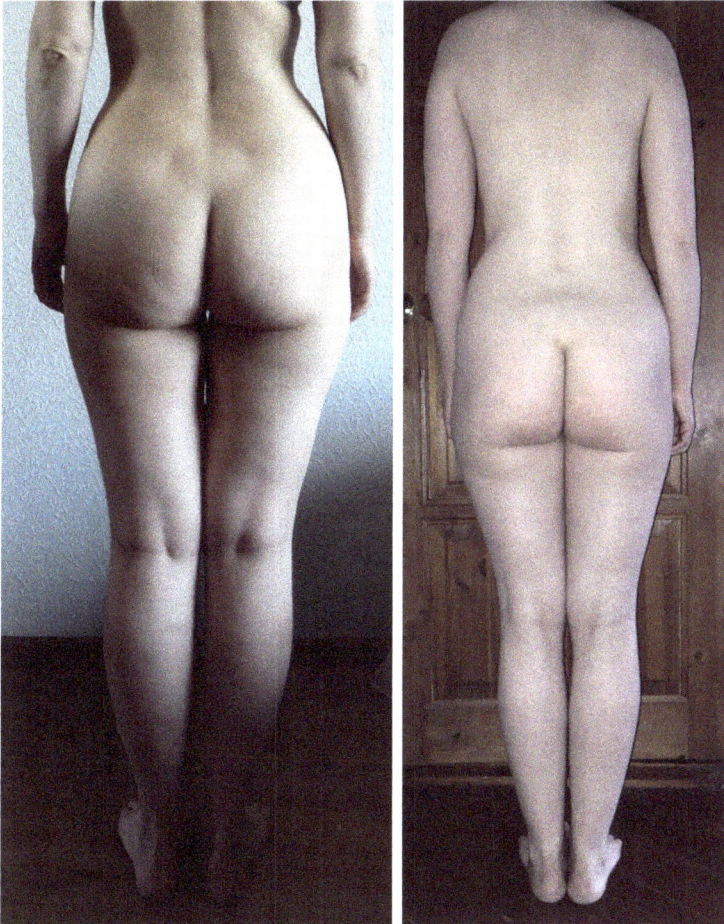

Gynecoid morphology, psoric miasm. The woman on the left is a gravida 2, has hypothyroidism. The woman on the right is gravida 1, no chronic health problems. They gave birth normally at home with no complications.

midwife it is usually a pleasure to work with such a woman, as her level of second-circle presence allows the birth team to trust her completely. She tends to understand recommendations well. She prefers working as a team and avoids conflicts. She has a strong ability (and desire) to trust and indeed can be overly trusting at times. She tries to follow the midwife's recommendations diligently and do everything so that the baby is born healthy. On the less positive side, she does not always do well with changes in plans. However, if potential problems are discussed ahead of time, with a detailed explanation of alternate plans and potential outcomes, she is usually able to adapt well. For the midwife it helps to understand that feeling safe is of prime importance for this woman. She blossoms in the warmth of a reassuring atmosphere.

The gynecoid-psoric woman tends to have problems absorbing nutrients from her food, even when she eats a nutritious diet. The vital force of this type tends to find resolution to deeper problems by throwing symptoms out to the surface: these women tend to have skin eruptions of all kinds, and more frequent discharges in the form of colds, eye and ear inflammation, sore throats, and other mild acute illnesses. Their digestion is slow and they tend toward constipation. Circulation is also generally slower and during pregnancy we observe more varicose veins and hemorrhoids among this type than others.

The pear-shaped morphology of a gynecoid woman is reflective of her attachment to the earth: her hips are wider, more voluminous, and heavier than her shoulders, and therefore her body is as if counterbalanced toward the earth. Her body walks on the earth like a bell, collecting all the earthly energy to itself through the sacrum and giving it back. Postpartum the gynecoid-psoric woman appreciates and is improved by emotional support from her caregivers and loved ones. She tends toward emotional ups and downs and becomes quite distraught if support is not forthcoming. She is a very attentive and loving mother and has no desire to cut breastfeeding short, for example.

Of the other miasms encountered with the gynecoid morphology, the tubercular and cancer miasms are most frequently observed. A tubercular gynecoid woman would tend to be more slender and often quite svelte, with the accompanying thin bone mass and fine features. A large percentage of gynecoid women in Russia are of this type. They seem to have nowhere to carry a baby within their slight frame. As the pregnancy advances, they seem to become "all baby," toting large round bellies without a hint of edema. They birth with ease and rarely suffer lacerations. Gynecoid women of the cancer miasm are more commonly average to slender body build. Many such women choose to give birth at home, reflecting the earth-mother qualities of the cancer miasm.

Men with gynecoid morphology, in spite of it being called the "female" pelvis, are in the majority, just as women. Their morphology can be surmised by looking at the rhombus, the relationship of the legs to each other, the shoulder slope, the relation of the shoulders to the hips, the shape and size of the hands and fingers, feet and toes, the dental arch, and so on—just as in the woman.

Voice and Presence in a Gynecoid person

> ...So I, for fear of trust, forget to say
> the perfect ceremony of love's rite,
> and in mine own love's strength seem to decay,
> o'ercharged with burthen of mine own love's might...
> Shakespeare, Sonnet 23

A person of gynecoid morphology and psoric miasm often has, or has had in the past, many insecurities, as stated above. These insecurities center around feeling safe. The degree to which such an individual feels safe as an adult is greatly determined by the environment of childhood. This miasmatic-morphological type needs to know that survival is assured. If such a child is sent off to daycare early, or if the mother begins working full time when the child is an infant, this person becomes withdrawn into first circle. Such a child will develop a fear of interacting with adults or with strangers (misanthropy), fear of going to school, fear of trying anything new, fear of going to camps or activities without a parent. The main strategy for a person of this type is to become "seen and not heard." They demonstrate extreme attachment to, and fear of losing, the parents, and express their affection. They will attempt to increase the parents' love for them by being well-behaved, but not to the point of fastidiousness like the cancer miasm. Doing well in school would be a good strategy for increasing parental attention, but the psoric type must work hard to become an excellent student. Things don't always come easy for them but when motivated by the need for love, they are "slow but steady" like the tortoise. They don't choose acts of bravado as a means of receiving attention, the way their android counterparts might; fighting is too threatening for them and they will only do so if pushed by their group of support. They are not risk-takers. On the other hand they are sensitive, kind, compassionate, and very trusting if given the slightest indication that it is safe to do so.

All of these factors combine to encourage, in difficult circumstances, a tightening of the throat and breathing high in the chest rather than low in the pelvis. This happens when a person of this type wants to express some feeling but suppresses it out of fear. There could be an actual deficit of attention and/or affection, but it is equally important to consider the intrinsic sensitivity of this particular miasmatic type for whom even slight deficits might be interpreted as severe.

In such children we observe frequent problems in the throat area: laryngitis, tonsillitis, chronic (recurring) sore throat, hoarseness, or a sensation of a lump in the throat (*globus hystericus*). If such a decompensated child or young adult experiences deep grief, and has the susceptibility, they can develop autoimmune thyroiditis, specifically thyrotoxicosis or Graves' disease. One study examined four children who developed Graves': in three of the patients the trigger event was represented by bereavement after death of a close relative; in the fourth case the boy's loss was enforced in traumatic separation from his mother figure. In all these children, depression was the common response to loss. The observed relationship between the affective disturbance and Graves' disease is compatible with one or more hypothetical models. One such pathway, via depletion of brain monoamines associated with the state of depression, could cause an activation of the hypothalamic-pituitary-adrenal axis with resultant suppression of immune surveillance. This could permit the formation of thyroid-stimulating immunoglobulins (TSI) and hence Graves' disease in genetically susceptible (HLA B-8) persons.[34] To cope with physical and/or psychological threats, the human body activates multiple processes, mediated by a close interconnection among brain, endocrine and inflammatory systems. Another study assessed the hypothalamic-pituitary-adrenal (HPA) and hypothalamic-pituitary-thyroid (HPT) axes' involvement after an acute stressful event (in this instance the Emilia Romagna earthquake swarm that occurred in northern Italy in 2012) and confirmed a recruitment of HPT axis after stressful events, together with increased incidence of altered TSH. This study increased understanding about the connection between external stressors and endocrine regulation[35].

In working with voice and presence, trained voice coaches have no difficulty identifying whether the breath is low and the throat open. In the gynecoid-psoric person who has had some emotional suppression, we can observe a difficulty in keeping the breath down and the voice low. Performing exercises to get the breath down often stimulates tears or emotional release. This type of person does not have trouble being present in second circle. Coming into eye contact and connecting with others is not the difficulty. Remaining in a state of connection while using the voice and breath, however, is emotionally overwhelming and so what we observe might be an unnaturally high voice (in a woman it could be a falsetto, as is commonly observed in many Russian women). Exercises that can help this group of people include:

---

34   Morillo E, Gardner LI. (1979). "Bereavement as an antecedent factor in thyrotoxicosis of childhood: four case studies with survey of possible metabolic pathways." *Psychosom Med.* Nov;41(7):545-55. doi: 10.1097/00006842-197911000-00005. PMID: 395558.

35   Spaggiari G, Setti M, Tagliavini S, Roli L, De Santis MC, Trenti T, Rochira V, Santi D. (2021). "The hypothalamic-pituitary-adrenal and -thyroid axes activation lasting one year after an earthquake swarm: results from a big data analysis." *J Endocrinol Invest.* Jul;44(7):1501-1513.

- Lots of practice reciting emotionally difficult texts;
- Deep squatting, keeping the heels on the floor, while speaking a text;
- Crawling on the floor and lifting each leg high from the hip, while speaking text or intoning vowels;
- Energetic movement during and between lines of text;
- Speaking text in a softer, lower voice but with breath low in the pelvis.

The aim of such exercises is to facilitate overcoming the person's fear to trust—not so much trusting others, as the self. He or she must practice repeatedly until there is more comfort expressing feelings. A hand placed gently on the lower back while the person is speaking is welcomed by this type of individual and can be used generously until a place of security in the self is achieved.

CHAPTER SEVEN.

Android Morphology

A discussion about android morphology is best begun by describing the numerous physical and physiological nuances characteristic of this type. Android morphology presents a completely different totality from that of gynecoid or any other type and is most often observed in a mixed form (gynecoid-android or android-gynecoid being the most common mix). It is perhaps the most *potentially* complication-ridden morphological type because of specific characteristics which may influence labor or general health.

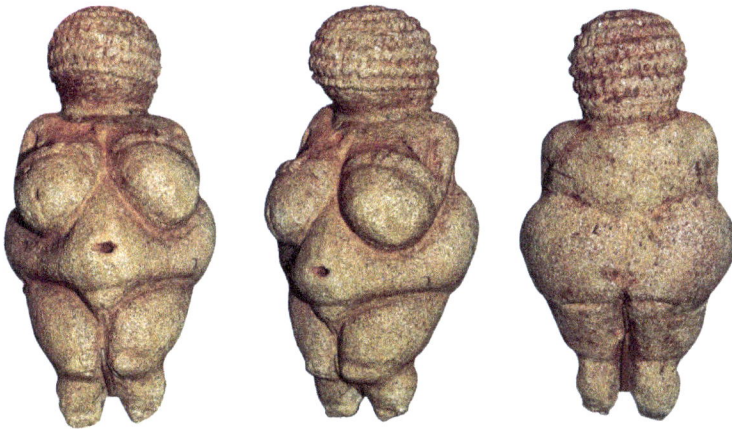

Android morphology is typified in the "Venus of Willendorf". Venus of Willendorf, also called Woman of Willendorf or Nude Woman, Upper Paleolithic female figurine found in 1908 at Willendorf, Austria, that is perhaps the most familiar of some 40 small portable human figures (mostly female) that had been found intact or nearly so by the early 21st century.
Kuiper, Kathleen. "Venus of Willendorf". Encyclopedia Britannica, 11 Jul. 2018, https://www.britannica.com/topic/Venus-of-Willendorf. Accessed 1 May 2021.

The android morphology has been historically known as the "male pelvis," although this term is far from accurate, insofar as men can possess any morphological type just as women can. The android shape is also referred to as the "apple", or the inverted triangle, with the sharp point at the feet. Women of this morphology are more massive on the top, with large chests or breasts, a wide waistline, and gradually tapering legs which end in ankles disproportionately delicate in comparison with the woman's other features. The feet are on the small side. Such a morphological type is found in 32.5% of White women, and in 15.7% of non-White women. A very large number of android types are found in Europe and the UK.

The inlet of the android pelvis is heart-shaped. The back is wedge-shaped while the front is narrow and triangular. The posterior sagittal diameter is rather short in comparison with the anterior sagittal diameter, and the anterior side is narrowed. This means that the space in the anterior of the pelvis is very limited to accommodate the fetal occiput, forcing it to lie occiput-posterior. The excess weight carried around the middle creates the impression of a large baby, and in fact women with android morphology do have a tendency toward gestational diabetes (the android hyperandrogenous tendency also gives rise to insulin resistance and obesity).

The android pelvis has the shape of a funnel from top to bottom. The sacrum of an android woman is flat, and slopes toward the anterior the lower down it gets, which is why we observe comparatively small dimensions throughout. The pelvis is relatively deep owing to the massive bones. The sacrosciatic notch is narrow, with a high arch, measuring only 1.5–2 finger breadths. The walls of the pelvis are slightly convergent. The ischial spines are usually easily palpated and often protrude slightly into the pelvic cavity, thereby reducing the transverse dimension of the midpelvis. The pubic arch is narrow, less than 90°.

All in all, the anteroposterior diameter of an android pelvis is long, while the transverse diameter is short—just as in the anthropoid morphology, but the general morphological characteristics allows them to be easily differentiated (see the chapter on anthropoid morphology for a comparative table). This length in the anteroposterior size is reflected in the length of the perineum, which is also increased. What this means for birth is that there is actually more perineum for the baby to maneuver and the woman is more likely to have lacerations.

In search for evidence of the correlations between **morphology and hormones,** some very interesting studies have come to light. One study investigated the relationship between perineal length (what is termed anogenital distance or AGD) and endometriosis. The findings were fascinating not only for the predictability of such a daunting gynecological problem, but also in relation to ramifications for childbirth. The authors reported that

> In experimental models, AGD at birth reflects hormonal exposure during prenatal life and predicts AGD in adulthood (Dean et al, 2012, Hotchkiss et al, 2004, Macleod et al, 2010, Wolf et al, 2002, Wu et al, 2010). In animals, it is well established that more androgens results in longer AGD. Similarly, studies in human males have shown that association. Exposure to anti-androgens results in shorter (more feminine) AGD in infant males (Swan et al, 2005, Swan et al, 2015). The link between higher estrogen exposure in utero and shorter AGD (which would be our model here) has been reported by our group recently (Mendiola et al., 2016), and as far as we know has not yet been explored in other adult human studies. Evidence from animal models (Boberg et al, 2013, Christiansen et al, 2014) and human studies, however, have shown that maternal exposure to xenoestrogen substances, i.e., bisphenol A, phytoestrogens and monobutyl phthalate, reduces AGD in newborn females (Huang et al., 2009). Therefore, we hypothesized that AGD length is modulated by the intrauterine hormonal androgen–estrogen environmental milieu, and, consequently, it may be used as a surrogate and reliable biomarker of that prenatal hormonal environment.[36]

---

36 Maria L. Sánchez-Ferrer, et al. (2017), "Investigation of anogenital distance as a diagnostic tool in endometriosis." *Reproductive Biomedicine Online,* Volume 34, Issue 4, P375-382.

The investigators conclude that there is a correlation between *higher estrogen levels and shorter AGD, and, conversely, between longer AGD and higher androgen levels.* This is a sensational discovery because it immediately opens up a wellspring of hypotheses about morphological type and hormonally dependent conditions.

Needless to say, the length of a woman's perineum absolutely correlates with the diameters of her pelvic outlet, which in turn correlate with the pelvic diameters as a whole—that is, with her morphology. One element cannot be separated from the whole. What these authors attribute to a "prenatal hormonal environment" certainly can be extrapolated to embrace much more: any hormonal environment does not originate *in utero* (unless the woman is taking hormones) but is a specific expression of the morphological totality of that woman. Her morphology includes everything that makes her unique as a woman, and makes her similar to other women with a similar morphology. As indicated above, her "hormonal environment" is not only evidenced by her anogenital distance, but equally expressed in her weight distribution, face and jaw shape, bone mass, length and shape of arms, legs, fingers, and toes—and, yes, in her miasmatic/constitutional tendencies. Thus, any number of these elements when perceived as a whole can point to the same morphological type, for which there are very specific hormonal expressions, including (but not limited to) androgen dominance and estrogen under-expression. [37]

The most relevant goal is not to discover where a specific trait began, or what gave rise to it; linear cause-and-effect explanations are unhelpful and reductionistic and don't consider the totality of the person. The symptoms (or traits) of the pattern can be identified *in total*, and we regard it altogether as actualization of specific soul-intent, entelechy laid out before us. This is extremely important to grasp. Recognizing

---

37   Azziz R., Carmina E., Dewailly D., Diamanti-Kandarakis E., Escobar-Morreale H.F., Futterweit W., Janssen O.E., Legro R.S., Norman R.J., Taylor A.E., Witchel S.F. (2006). "Androgen Excess Society, Positions statement: criteria for defining polycystic ovary syndrome as a predominantly hyperandrogenic syndrome: an Androgen Excess Society guideline." *J. Clin. Endocrinol. Metab.;* 91: 4237-4245.

the unique characteristics of each morphological type makes us more sensitive observers and more helpful practitioners. On the other hand, hormonal-morphological connections should not be reduced to black and white interpretations. As several authors of one study concluded, "Traditional views whereby sexual dimorphisms between women and men are explained almost exclusively by the presence of estrogens in women and androgens in men must be modified to reflect the complexities of steroid hormone signaling and biology."[38] Reducing men and women to a mixture of hormones is just as one-sided as any other reductionist reasoning. We're not interested in supposed causes because there are none. There are only individual souls in the process of becoming—physically, mentally, emotionally. What interests us is how to identify barriers to this becoming and help people to overcome them.

Android women and men have a pronounced jaw, often squarish in shape. They have a large build and square shoulders. The waist is wide and takes on weight first. The hips are narrow, with a flat sacrum giving rise to flat buttocks and a low buttocks crease. Both men and women tend to develop "love handles." While clothed, an android woman seems to have voluminous hips due to the massiveness of the bones. Sometimes the android morphology can be recognized by the characteristic hands and feet: hands are wide in diameter, and fingers are short and square.

Since the pelvis has a funnel shape, the acetabulae angle downward and inward, making the trochanters relatively closely spaced and the thighs closely aligned and touching each other down to the knee when the woman stands with feet together, giving the legs an "x" shape. From the knee down the legs diverge. The android pelvis has a reduced pelvic tilt. This combination of factors logically results in thighs being quite close together and calves being angled outward in order to maintain balance. People with such morphology often cannot stand with their feet together without having to bend one knee ("knock-kneed"). People of

---

38   Stephen R. Hammes and Ellis R. Levin. (2019). "Impact of estrogens in males and androgens in females." *American Society for Clinical Investigation*, Volume 129, Issue 5. J Clin Invest. 2019;129(5):1818–1826.

this morphological type tend to "lock the knees," or at least seemingly do, and their knees often appear hyperextended. It is important to understand that such a stance is usually not consciously chosen, but is genetically inherited as part of a specific morphological totality. It is a morphological characteristic, undoubtedly interconnected with all the other traits of such a morphology.

The rhombus of an android woman is barely visible to the naked eye even after bearing children. Once the boundaries are identified with the fingers, it displays a very long vertical section and a short horizontal crossbar which is closer to the upper half of the rhombus. Locating the dimples with the fingers is challenging.

Locking the knees, in voice and presence work, is strongly discouraged; it is associated with tension in the body (and mind), blocked breath, and difficulty in responding in the here and now. In the martial arts, people are taught to bear their weight on the balls of the feet and keep the center of gravity forward in the body. Such a stance allows one to be constantly on the ready. The knees are necessarily slightly bent in such a position because locking them would not allow the center of gravity to be forward and would inhibit action. This is the stance of intention. It is the position of maximum presence and attention. Birthing women intuitively choose such positions as labor intensifies, and they begin to assume the hands-and-knees pose, or lean slightly forward while standing, bending the knees and dipping into a mild squat during contractions. The rhombus of Michaelis, as the visual part of the sacrum or energetic center of the physical body, rises up and dominates, becoming the fulcrum.

Locking the knees and walking not with the weight on the balls of the feet, but on the heels, is characteristic of third-circle energy. The third circle is that of domination, aggression; in third circle the person occupies all the space in the room. He or she talks with a loud, unpleasant voice—at nobody in particular (what Stanislavsky[39] referred to, in relation to actors, as "acting in general"). People who adopt such a stance

---

39   Konstantin Stanislavsky (1863-1938), Russian father of modern acting.

as their everyday pattern of interacting with the world are hard to be around for very long. Such a woman, during a prenatal visit or a homeopathic consultation, talks nonstop, jumps from one topic to the next, rarely makes eye contact but instead tends to look above people's heads. She doesn't seem to hear what the practitioner is saying. One becomes tired in the presence of third-circle energy.

Locked knees literally block one from connecting with others (and even with oneself). Try it for yourself: stand with your knees severely locked or as hyperextended as possible, and attempt to breathe low in your abdomen. It is nearly impossible. The breath is forced up, the connection with the earth is lost; the reflexive areas of the throat and cervix are disconnected. Yet such a stance, for most people of android morphology, is automatic. The questions that need to be asked are: is there a physiological explanation for this knee-locking in people of android morphology? And from the other direction: do we observe more third-circle energy among those with android morphology? If the first question has a plausible answer, then it follows that we would observe more third-circle behavior in people of android morphology. Indeed, this is the case. This conclusion ought not to be limiting, but freeing: imagine how much more constructive presence work can be done with people once we are able to diagnose their morphological type. Constitution, dominant miasms, morphology, and circle of attention—all these things are inherited *tendencies* which can be identified by the sensitive homeopath or the curious midwife or the insightful voice coach. These insights are ever so much more valuable than merely blaming everything on one's attitude or on one's psychological state (including traumatic events of the past), because it gives us material with which to work. It underscores the idea that people don't often assume their life stance consciously, but rather as a reflection of an overall adaptive mechanism that includes every other trait they are born with. It places less blame on the individual for being the master of her own fate and elicits compassion. It gives people something that they can understand, that they can consciously work on. It's all a reflection of one's *tropos*—the path or way each person is given as the means to realization of their divine image, or personal *logos*. We are all challenged, each in our individual way.

Whenever we observe a symptom—that is, a characteristic of the person which individualizes and differentiates from other people—we ask ourselves the question: what is this characteristic compensating for? Any symptom shrouds its opposite expression, for which it—what we observe—is the compensation reaction. Newton's third law is observed in all of nature and is the explanation behind why homeopathy works: for every action there is an equal and opposite reaction. An excessive capacity for movement shrouds a certain lack of stability and the body compensates by freezing up, contracting, going into spasm. The more severe the hypermobility, the more severe the compensatory spasms.

Hypermobile joints are defined as those that typically move beyond the normally accepted ranges of motion, taking into consideration age, sex, and ethnic background. The maximal range of movement that a joint is capable of is determined by the degree of tightness of the restraining ligaments. If a person locks the knees habitually, it means that she *can*. The primary cause of hypermobility is ligament laxity. Epidemiological studies have determined that hypermobility is seen in up to 10% of individuals in Western populations and as high as 25% in other populations. Joint hypermobility tends to run in families. The genetic conditions reflecting severe joint hypermobility most commonly reported in the literature are Ehlers-Danlos and Marfan syndrome. There is however a larger percentage of the population that has joint hypermobility not associated with a specific gene.

Joint hypermobility is a term used to describe excess joint movement. However, when joint hypermobility leads to symptoms in joints or other areas of the body, it is called benign joint hypermobility syndrome (BJHS). The characteristics of BJHS involve proprioception impairment, increased frequency of pain within joints and the tendency to injure soft tissues while performing physical activities. Most papers in the literature relating to joint hypermobility discuss this form. It might be suspected if the person easily sprains ankles or has had several fractures or traumas in their history.

Android Morphology

Joint strength is dependent upon the supporting ligament structure that crosses the joint space. Ligaments are composed mainly of collagen, the main component of connective tissue and the most abundant protein in the body, making up between 25% and 35% of the whole-body protein content. It is mostly found in fibrous tissues such as tendons, ligaments, and skin. Collagen tissues may be rigid, as in bones, compliant as in tendons, or have a gradient from stiff to flexible as in cartilage. Collagen is also abundant in the tissues of blood vessels, the digestive tract, inter-vertebral discs and viscera. In muscle tissue, collagen makes up about 6% of the tissue serving as a major component of the endomysium, the tissue that sheaths each individual muscle fiber. The fibroblast is the most common cell that creates collagen and plays a critical role in tissue repair and wound healing.[40] This information immediately provides us with a lengthy list of potential constitutional traits related to lowered levels of collagen. Whether as homeopaths or midwives (or other prac-titioners) our attention is drawn to what we observe in clinical practice among people of android morphology. We often see such symptoms as: flaccid skin, reduced muscle tone, constipation, and back pain (and often a history of disc problems).

Experience of midwives shows that women of android morphology have some form of hip dysplasia in their own history more frequently than any other morphological group, and are also the most common morphological type to give birth to babies with hip dysplasia. Thus far there is a glaring paucity of research correlating hip dysplasia (or benign joint hypermobility) with morphological type. Hip dysplasia in babies is also known to be more commonly associated with breech presentation. The midwifery/obstetric and neonatal specialties however have over-looked the fact that hip dysplasia and breech presentation are connected by the same factor—ligament laxity, and that these symptoms are most common in android morphology. Connections have been observed

---

40   Peter N. Fysh, DC, FICCP. (2018). "Benign joint hypermobility—developing clinical significance." *Journal of clinical chiropractic paediatrics*, Volume 17, No. 2, July.

between hip dysplasia and hypermobility, however,[41] which, as has already been shown, is a common trait in android women. Pulling all the elements together into a whole is what has been lacking.

Assessment of Joint Hypermobility

The most widely used method of joint hypermobility assessment is known as the Beighton score. The person is asked to perform a standard set of maneuvers and is given a score for each. The nine-point scale is based on the following assessments:

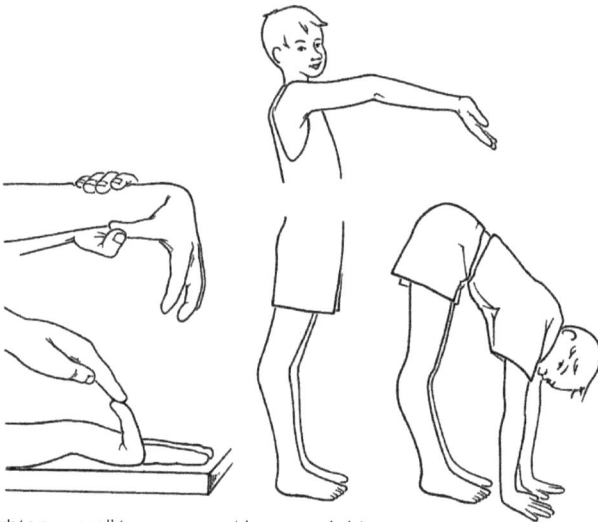

The "Beighton-score" to assess joint hypermobility.
Passive apposition of the thumb to the flexor aspect of the forearm; one point for each hand.
Passive dorsiflexion of the little finger beyond 90° ; one point for each hand.
Hyperextension of the elbow beyond 10°; one point for each elbow.
Hyperextension of the knees beyond 10°, one point for each knee.
Forward flexion of the trunk with the knees fully extended so that the palms of the hand rest flat on the floor; one point.
(Figure drawn by Susanne Staubli, University Children's Hospital, Zurich.)

---

41   Muldoon, M., Gosey, G., Healey, R., & Santore, R. (2016). "Hypermobility: a key factor in hip dysplasia. A prospective evaluation of 266 patients." Journal of Hip Preservation Surgery, 3(Suppl 1), hnw030.034.

1. passive apposition of the thumbs to touch the flexor aspect of the forearm,
2. passive dorsiflexion of the 5th fingers beyond $90°$,
3. hyperextension of the elbows beyond $10°$,
4. hyperextension of the knees beyond $10°$, and
5. ability to place the palms of both hands flat on the floor, with knees in extension.

The maximum score is 9. A score of 4 or greater confirms the classification of hypermobility. The score does not indicate specific areas of hypermobility within the body but is general in nature.

The android morphology is not by any means the only one to display a tendency toward joint hypermobility. It is also not infrequently observed in persons of anthropoid, and less frequently gynecoid, morphology. Hip dysplasia in babies however is rarely observed in those whose mothers are gynecoid, and when observed in a baby whose mother is anthropoid, is of the type that expresses inadequate bone formation. More about the expression of joint hypermobility is discussed in the chapter on the anthropoid morphology.

Android morphology and miasms

This morphological type is most often associated with the following miasms: psora, sycosis, or a syco-syphilitic mix. When associated with the sycotic miasm, we see the sycotic themes of growth, increase, and progress. If the psoric miasm is rooted in carving out a life that is safe, predictable, and reliable, the sycotic miasm is about making a life that is comfortable, financially secure, and successful in the eyes of the world. Psoric people tend to live most of their lives in first circle, withdrawn from others, concentrated on the past. Sycotics on the other hand tend to be third-circle people, the assertive overachievers out to achieve material comfort and look good while doing so.

The sycotic android woman is a sensitive, emotional person who does not always show her feelings. She is a reliable, responsible, hardworking, practical woman who often likes to be a leader in the family or at work. She is a devoted partner in marriage, has "a good head on her shoulders" and can be stubborn. She likes to make decisions herself. She is pragmatic, down to earth, and focused on the material well-being of her family; sometimes this is expressed by the fact that she seeks to have the best of everything. Sycotic constitutions are overly concerned about the opinions of others and how they look, and therefore they are constantly putting on what they regard as their ideal front. They want others to think highly of them. This makes them rather closed and sometimes artificial. External appearances become more important than vulnerable authenticity. They are pedantic and scrupulous about doing things the "right" way. Order and rules give them a sense of stability and predictability. In this regard they are often quite religious, sometimes extremely so, and their religiousness is based in the need to do everything right, which in turn is motivated by the desire to be seen doing everything right—so as to be loved. They need and like order. When android morphology and sycosis are combined, we see an anxious woman who tries to keep her feelings contained but tends to run her family like a navy ship.

Among the homeopathic constitutional types that most closely reflect this combination, are the *potassium salts:* Kali carbonicum, Kali sulphuricum, Kali phosphoricum, Kali arsenicosum, and, especially, Causticum. In the latter remedy we also find perhaps the highest frequency of hip dysplasia and joint hypermobility, compensated for by spasms, sometimes to the point of paralysis. This group is more *dogmatic* than it is materialistic (**Mind; dictatorial; dogmatic**: ars camph CAUST chlam-t FERR ***ferr-acet*** impa-w kali-br KALI-C lach lyc merc nux-v oxyg querc-r sep ***stoi-k*** thuj) and is concerned about the *family or group*, especially in regard to *justice, human rights, fairness, and the misuse of power by people in authority*. They are serious homemakers and conscientious parents who often go against the grain of society. They can be very *suspicious*, especially concerning others' financial motives (reflecting the sycotic obsession with creating a materially comfortable life on earth).

Their feelings reflect the polar opposites of both extreme *compassion* and *hard-heartedness*. They are *rigid* and don't do well with a change of plan. They are overly responsible and anxious. They are all very concerned with *doing the right thing.*

Other characteristic android-sycotic homeopathic remedy types include Natrum muriaticum (reserved; fastidious; tending toward hidden grief); Thuja (history of abuse and/or dysfunctional relationship with her mother; sees herself as fragile; desires everything beautiful); Lachesis (talkative, suspicious, sensual and creative leader with many fears). Remedies like Sepia, Pulsatilla, Phosphorus, Silicea, Carcinosinum, Arsenicum album, Ignatia, Lycopodium, Nux vomica are rarely associated with android morphology of any miasm. Android-psoric homeopathic constitutional types include any of the carbon salts: Calcarea carbonicum, Ammonium carbonicum, Magnesium carbonicum, Graphites, Carbo vegetabilis, Borax.

An android woman can do without the presence of her husband during childbirth and sometimes even prefers it. During birth she does not become emotionally dependent, but will be very grateful to the midwife for her active support. Android-sycotic women might choose home birth because they consider it a superior option, or because it is a fashion among her friends; or because they are suspicious of doctors and hospitals. That is, she cares about the correct-

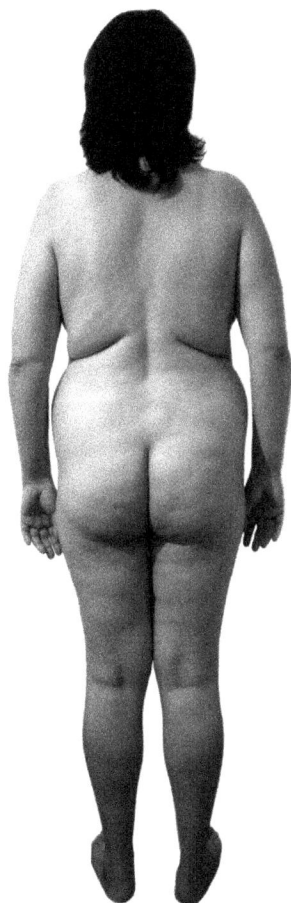

Characteristic android morphology. This woman had a lengthy first labor but later gave birth to another 5 children precipitously at home in under one hour.

ness of such a choice. She appreciates professionalism, as it is always important for her how others perceive her, and so she will choose caregivers who excel in their field or have a lot of experience. So long as you have her trust and she is not suspect of your authority, working with such women is usually a positive experience. Their dogmatic, rigid side can sometimes complicate the relationship if they aren't prepared ahead of time for what could happen; therefore, it is wise to discuss such possibilities in detail and make a feasible alternative plan.

Labor

Android women (especially primiparae) have a higher incidence of labor complications, most of all since their babies tend to occupy the occiput-posterior position. It has always been explained that this is due to lack of space in the posterior part of the pelvis. In light of the high frequency of joint hypermobility and potential laxity of ligaments in android women, however, this too may be an important factor in the baby's "inability" to settle down into the pelvis.

In an android primiparous woman we can expect the baby to drop into the pelvis late, or not until labor. Therefore, we frequently find that the baby's sinciput rides above the pubic bone until the first stage of labor, making the baby seem large for gestational age. The woman often complains of symphysitis during the last weeks and perhaps lower back pain. If her joint hypermobility is extreme, she may experience an unusually wide separation of the pubic symphysis.

Often these primiparous women begin laboring only well after their due date and frequently their labors are induced. The labor is very frequently preceded by premature rupture of the membranes, which is often observed in association with occiput-posterior babies, whose heads exert uneven pressure on the cervix and the bony pelvis. In addition, the possible collagen deficit in these women would contribute to more friable membranes. Her insulin resistance and tendency toward gestational diabetes might lead to a chronic yeast infection during pregnancy, which further works to weaken the integrity of the amniotic sac. If her bag of waters breaks before contractions start and she is nearing or past 42 weeks' gestation, the likelihood of the baby passing meconium before labor starts is greatly increased, thus revealing greenish stained fluid. Such a situation is a midwife's nightmare, insofar as the baby is already showing signs of possible placental insufficiency, is occiput-posterior, and the mother has a likely unripe cervix—and still has the entire labor ahead. Without a doubt, prevention is the best cure for the complications encountered in android primiparae. This is not the absolute fate of every android first-time mother, but it would be unprofessional of the midwife to ignore the morphological signs during the prenatal period and not make recommendations to prevent such a scenario from developing. Early passage of moderate meconium before onset of contractions in a primiparous woman is an indication to transfer to hospital; if the baby is indeed posterior and large, cesarean section is usually the optimal route of delivery to avoid hypoxia and meconium aspiration and all the possible sequelae those imply.

Assuming though that the fluid is clear, and contractions have commenced, there is a characteristic course of labor in android women. The funnel shape of the android pelvis means that the baby might descend rather quickly in active labor up until it reaches the narrow part of the "funnel." At that point (usually at 7 cm dilation or so) the head must now mold considerably in order to navigate the narrowing cavity and outlet. This, combined with the most common posterior presentation, makes for a long and painful first stage. The woman (and indeed the midwife) are encouraged after the first vaginal exam, when labor has not been going on so long at all and her cervix is already well dilated, only to find that the work has just begun.

Due to the insulin resistance seen in these women, the babies are usually large, which further intensifies the challenges. The baby's head being occiput-posterior means that molding and very intense contractions are required in order for it to be brought down onto the pelvic floor, where it will make its internal rotation into the occiput-anterior position at the very last minute. These things can be rushed with the addition of synthetic uterotonics like oxytocin (in a hospital setting, as they are contraindicated in an out-of-hospital setting) but they are often not called for. With a holistic, accurate understanding of the woman's morphology, the midwife should be reassured that such a labor is par for the course. Occiput-posterior labors don't have to be regarded as pathological. Although they tend to be longer and more painful, they are nevertheless a variation of normal. On the other hand, wisdom dictates that prevention is the best cure, and prevention of labor dystocia for the android primipara entails recommending evening primrose oil starting at 24 weeks' gestation—to facilitate timely ripening of the cervix. This simple recommendation is very effective at preventing postmaturity and its attendant problems. Exercises, the aim of which is to convince the baby to turn into an anterior position, are however useless.

The baby does not choose that position in any kind of a conscious manner. All kinds of midwives' tales have been concocted in different places and different eras to explain why a baby is posterior in labor (and then various methods have been devised to explain these "reasons"). Knowing that her morphological type most likely includes ligament laxity, we can infer that the baby, as "passenger" through this maternal vessel, is exposed to perhaps less-than-average resistance from the muscle fibers of the woman's uterus and abdomen. Android women with posterior babies should not feel that they need to "do something about it" before labor. The baby did not get confused, and the mother did not do anything wrong. She has android morphology with more or less of its attendant characteristics and predispositions. The fact of the matter is: nearly all occiput-posterior babies turn spontaneously into the anterior position when the head reaches the pelvic floor and they are born naturally with no pathological ramifications (see chapter 10: Morphology and Occiput-Posterior Birth). Our job as midwives is to help the mother prevent the development of gestational diabetes (which would mean a large baby) and going well past her due date (in a primiparous woman). Both of these can be achieved and therefore her risks can be reduced.

While android women often suffer from ligament laxity (and the more so during pregnancy in connection with changes in the hormonal mix, including especially the increases in progesterone and relaxin), their musculature, interestingly, displays a kind of thickness not common among the other morphological types. This is noted from the first prenatal visit, and later as the baby grows and the midwife has difficulty palpating its position. It's not only explained by the excess fat carried around the middle but also by thicker than average muscles. The long perineum, together with a slightly reduced transverse diameter of the pelvic outlet, increases the mother's likelihood of tears as the head is emerging. In a primipara, the perineum seems to be pulled downward and outward together with the head. Tears can be avoided if the head is allowed to stretch the perineal muscles gradually.

Android women don't always have trouble giving birth. If the total pelvic volume is adequate in relation to the thickness of the bones, the prognosis should be good. Estimated baby weight and gestational age also influence prognosis. We consider all factors collectively. For example, if the woman is a first-time mother and her transverse diameter of the rhombus is 10 cm, the Soloviev index is 16.5 cm, and the estimated weight of the baby at 39 weeks is 4 kg, a good prognosis is far from guaranteed, since she has heavy bone mass and the "plane of least dimensions" is minimal. With such a woman, we should do everything in our power— within the framework of safety—to facilitate the birth of the baby by the expected date of birth. Having studied her morphology early in pregnancy, we would recommend evening primrose oil from the 24th week to increase the likelihood of the body making optimal hormonal preparation to give birth by the estimated due date. We would also recommend strict dietary restrictions: the exclusion of all sweet and starchy foods, including the limitation of sweet fruits, so that the baby does not grow too large and the pregnant woman does not develop gestational diabetes.

The android morphology represents an exception to the rule that in all primiparae, the baby should engage by one week before the birth for a good prognosis. In the case of android women, we make a prediction more on the basis of the condition of the cervix: its ripeness, i.e., location in the lower uterine segment; its softness and flexibility; and most of all its degree of effacement. Even in the case of premature rupture of the membranes we must first take into account the condition of the cervix in order to predict the course of labor. For example, if the cervix is completely effaced at the moment of spontaneous rupture, we calmly wait for the commencement of contractions and a normal course of labor.

Android multiparae have their own peculiarity: the preliminary phase can last a long time, due to the posterior position of the baby and the funnel-shaped form of the pelvis. During this period, the baby adapts to the pelvis and comes into the optimal position. Do not rush if the laboring woman feels good and is able to rest. Often the membranes rupture during the preliminary phase. The baby's head during this period will be at a high station, and the sagittal suture will be either oblique or in the transverse diameter—lying, as it were, above the pelvic brim.

With normal dimensions, the multiparous android woman gives birth slowly at the beginning, and then the process picks up speed quickly and unexpectedly after the baby conforms to the pelvis. Usually he turns into an anterior position at the very last moment, after which he is born in 1–3 contractions. This internal rotation of the head is clearly visible from the outside, and is often "announced" by a sudden trickle of amniotic fluid. Due to the fact that the multiparous android woman may not pay much attention to the contractions of the preliminary period, she sometimes gives birth at home alone, when contractions are unexpectedly intensified and the baby suddenly descends onto the pelvic floor in one contraction, and is born with the next. For this reason, such a woman should be prepared so that she can recognize the preliminary contractions and call her midwives as soon as the process has begun; and her midwives should not wait but try to arrive at her home within a short time.

The newborn of an android woman should always be carefully checked for hip dysplasia and referred to an orthopedist if the characteristic "click" is detected on examination. Torticollis is another condition

Android Morphology

more commonly observed in newborns of android mothers. It should be emphasized again that such conditions are hardly ever the result of birth trauma, but rather manifest as constitutional expressions. These conditions can be treated homeopathically and often do not necessitate treatment from a chiropractor or osteopath. Both of these latter modalities tend to antidote homeopathic treatment, and so the parents should be informed as to this incompatibility and make their decisions accordingly.

Cases

Case 1: Teresa

Theresa came to see me for a consultation after her first pregnancy and birth had been fraught with complications. As she began telling the story of how she had gone into labor but contractions never really became strong and her doctor had decided to augment with oxytocin, I made note of her android features. She had the characteristic inverted triangle body shape, with shoulders wider than her hips comparatively. Her bust was on the large side. Her wrists and ankles though were quite delicate looking. The form of her legs revealed a slight x-shape from hip to heel.

When she was young, a gynecologist had told her she would never have any children. Making the connection with her morphology, I immediately asked whether she had been diagnosed with polycystic ovarian syndrome, and she concurred that, yes, this indeed had been blamed for her assumed infertility.

She reported that after a long labor with unbearably strong, artificially induced contractions, she had finally reached a fully dilated cervix, but the baby was not descending well. Her birth care providers had orchestrated active pushing during each contraction. She said that the doctor had her hand continuously in her vagina, apparently trying to manipulate the baby's head, and at the same time was exerting pressure on her pelvic floor muscles in order to stimulate her urge to push. This had been exhausting and, after 90 minutes, unsuccessful, as the baby had not descended sufficiently and at this point was showing signs of stress. It was decided to perform a cesarean section. Her baby was born weighing 4450 grams (9 lbs 8 oz) with Apgar scores of 7 and 8.

She wasn't so bothered by the fact of the operation as much as she was by what happened after: within a day or so she began experiencing excruciating lower back pain. The pain could not be alleviated with pain medication. Eventually she had an MRI performed and it was found that she had two herniated discs in her lumbar spine. Theresa made the conclusion that this spinal trauma had been caused by the doctor's manipulations during labor.

I completed a thorough morphological exam, and explained to Theresa what I was observing along the way. Noting that Theresa had scored the maximum 9 points on the Beighton assessment for hyper-mobility, I told her that this had most probably been connected with the herniated discs during birth, and that this symptom is part of a morpho-logical totality that also often includes polycystic ovaries and gestational diabetes, as well as posterior position of the baby during labor—all factors which contributed to her complicated birth.

Theresa was very relieved to have a more integrated picture of herself and her birth story. Now she was interested in preventing problems for her next pregnancy, and so she began homeopathic treat-ment after a full consultation.

Case 2: Alice

Alice came to me during her second pregnancy with a strong desire to give birth at home. The first birth, she said, was "just a nightmare," which she didn't want to repeat. During her first pregnancy she had been under the care of midwives and planned a home birth. But when the gestational age reached 43 weeks and she was repeatedly showing glucose in her urine, the midwives decided to send her to the hospital. Labor was initiated with oxytocin with an unripe cervix and a large baby.

Despite the low likelihood of a successful induction, Alice's labor progressed at a normal rate and she reached full dilation after about 8 hours. At this point the baby's head began its descent into the outlet very slowly. When the head was finally born three hours later, the baby's shoulders were stuck, and the obstetrician had to perform a large episiotomy and use every extreme measure to get the baby born. Alice's 4500-gram (9 lbs 9 oz) baby was born in a state of asphyxia, and she endured an extended laceration from the episiotomy into the rectum, amounting to a serious third-degree tear, from which she complained of continuing discomfort to this day.

Her morphological assessment revealed a typical android pelvis, with a transverse diameter of her rhombus measuring 9.5 cm, as well as massive bones, with a Soloviev index of 17 cm. Her pelvic outlet was narrow with an inter-tuberous diameter of 9 cm.

We discussed the connection between her morphology, her dominant miasm—in this case sycoto-syphilis, with strong feelings of anger, resentment, and blame—and made a care plan. The plan included work in acquiring the skills of presence, so that she could more readily take responsibility for her role in her own labors. She was determined to change her diet to help prevent gestational diabetes. An understanding of her morphology and constitutional trends was central to her being able and willing to accept what had already happened and move on.

After a healthy pregnancy, Alice went into labor spontaneously at 41 weeks and 3 days. The labor progressed smoothly until the last, but with the slowed birth of the head, the shoulders were a bit too broad to emerge gracefully. A quick change of position—moving from the birth stool into a squat—jiggled the baby in just the right way and he was born very quickly thereafter, weighing 4 kg (8 lbs 8 oz) and quite healthy.

Android Morphology

CHAPTER EIGHT.

Anthropoid Morphology

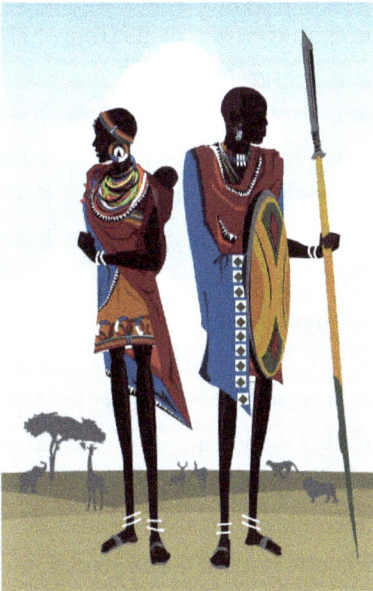

https://www.behance.net/
gallery/20600143/Maasai-Tribal-
Composition-Animation/modules/
138502027

According to a study of skeletal material carried out by Caldwell and Maloy in the 1930s, 40.5% of Blacks in the sample exhibited anthropoid pelvic types, whereas the frequency was just 23.5% in Whites.[42] By far it is most frequently observed in people of African descent. The anthropoid morphology is identified by finding a rhombus of Michaelis that is quite long in the anteroposterior diameter and relatively narrow in the transverse diameter. The characteristic anthropoid body type is seen among professional runners: they stand tall and straight as a tree, narrow from side to side when seen face-on, with developed gluteus maximus and leg muscles. Their faces are long and narrow as well. Such people can also be seen among the models on runways of elite fashion designers. People with this morphology are usually supple and graceful in their movements.

---

42   Caldwell, W.E, Maloy, H.C., and D'Esopo. (1936). "The Anthropoid Pelvis." *American Journal of Obstetrics and Gynecology,* 32:5 p. 727.

This pelvic shape got its name from its association, in the 19th century, with the so-called "ape pelvis,", which is very narrow in the transverse and long in the anteroposterior diameter. The head of this morphological type, when viewed from the side, displays a large, round occiput—being dolichocephalic, wider from front to back than from side to side. They have long necks and squared shoulders. Their shoulders are the same width or slightly wider than their hips. Their fingers are long, as are their toes, and they have large narrow feet. Possibly the ethnic group to exhibit this morphology most characteristically of all is the Maasai tribe of eastern Africa. From the Maasai we can learn a great deal about other attendant constitutional and miasmatic characteristics of this morphology. Therefore, it will be useful to use them as a prototype.

It should have become clear by this point that no symptom or characteristic can be removed from the totality. It is not logical to conclude that the tall stature of the Maasai, for example, is a consequence of their heavy milk consumption (and therefore calcium intake), as many have done. The more appropriate question is: why do the Maasai choose to live almost exclusively on milk and meat, and how is that attribute related to their morphology? To make the conclusion about their height based on their diet would be akin to ascribing the height of a giraffe to its consumption of tree leaves. When we look at a giraffe we don't question why it is so tall and lean; we only know that it is a giraffe, and has specific characteristics. These two elements—tall stature and milk and meat consumption—are both present and observable in the Maasai, but one does not originate in or cause the other. From the phenomenological homeopathic viewpoint, we make note of all observable symptoms and regard them as part of one picture. The tall stature, anthropoid morphology, high consumption (i.e., desire for) milk and meat all fit together into one holistic picture. There are no separate "causes" for any of these symptoms, but together they compose an image: a people, which is greater than the sum of its parts. Together with the aforementioned symptoms can be added their particular cultural traditions, like their *adumu* dance, the brilliantly dyed red and blue textiles they make for clothing, their pastoral-nomadic way of life, their particular style of body adornment, their adoration for their cows, their initiation and coming-of-age rituals, and so on.

The homeopath has no difficulty recognizing all of these symptoms as characteristic of the tubercular miasm. People having anthropoid morphology, in turn, usually have characteristic symptoms of the tubercular miasm. Tuberculosis, as an acute and subsequently a chronic disease, expresses itself in the lungs, the bones, or the central nervous system. Tuberculosis finds its soil in people who have lost their homes: during wartime, when the enemy attacks and destroys one's home; in refugee populations when people have been forced to flee from their home and are in search of a new one; in prisons (not so much due to the crowding as is usually reasoned based on the germ theory, but in association again with being away from home); in dire poverty where people dwell in dank spaces (more in connection with lack of a real home than with crowded spaces). The incidence of TB was highest during peak times of the Industrial Revolution. Poverty and sometimes famine brought migrants from rural areas into cities to fuel the revolution, where they worked long hours in inhumane conditions. Once again the common denominator is *displacement*.

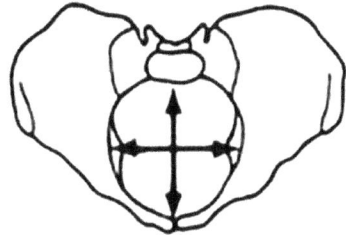

Anthropoid pelvis

The theme of the tubercular miasm is *the endless search*. We can take it farther and assert that this miasm is about losing (actually or symbolically) one's home and the anguish of then searching for it. People who come down with tuberculosis in our age of adequate sanitation and living spaces who are neither refugees nor prisoners do so because they are susceptible to the tubercular totality; we say, as homeopaths, that they are "tubercular." Tuberculosis is an excellent example of the shortcomings of the germ theory of infectious disease. Statistics for its frequency and death rate are barely more than 100 years old, yet they demonstrate a distinct connection with wars and displacement. The chronic expression of tubercular characteristics assumes the category of miasm.

People for whom this miasm is dominant are similar to those who suffer from acute TB: they are always making changes, in a state of constant flux; they are not content to "stay in one place." The homeopathic repertory gives these rubrics[43]: *Mind; change, desire for, constantly; Mind; change; desire for; surroundings;* and even *Generalities; weather; change of, desires!* Long-term stability is not a comfort for them but a limitation; it reeks for them of stagnation. They need their freedom (*Mind; freedom; desire for; Mind; domination by others aggravates.*). This is simply a psychological trait of the tubercular miasm. Such individuals might change their place of living many times during a lifetime, or, alternatively, change their occupation, their way of life, their convictions, their marriages. When a tubercular person is prevented from achieving change, it brings on apathy, moodiness, disappointment, and restlessness. Furthermore, these people have an inordinate desire to travel. Interestingly (and quite homeopathically), travel and change were actually prescribed for "consumptives in the 19th century. Not at all surprisingly, consumptive patients dominated the traveling invalid scene; in 1850, an estimated 90% of traveling British invalids suffered from consumption. The "change of air" was a 19th-century tourism form premised on the restoration of health.[44] Dr. James Lindsay, for example, in the mid-1800s, believed in removing the consumptive not just to a healthier climate but also "to an out-door life of healthful activity". More importantly, however, he maintained that the treatment of consumption required a "change of air, change of diet, change of scenery, change of daily routine, change involving the abandonment of many an injurious habit which has long been the secret minister of disease". Lindsay was convinced that this "great boon of change" benefited the consumptive more than any other aspect of the "change of air."[45] Such universally accepted methods of treatment for tuberculosis were,

---

43 Rubrics given in italics are taken from the Complete Dynamics online repertory and represent rubrics of the remedy *Tuberculinum*.

44 Richard E. Morris. (2018). "The Victorian 'change of air' as medical and social construction." *Journal of Tourism History*, DOI: 10.1080/1755182X.2018.1425485.

45 James Alexander Lindsay, *The Climatic Treatment Of Consumption: A Contribution Based on Medical Climatology* (London: MacMillan & Co. 1887).

without the field of medicine being consciously aware of it, homeopathically appropriate! The nomadism of the Maasai people further confirms their tubercular miasmatic basis.

In the depth of the tubercular soul the person seeks their spiritual home in God, and will never be satisfied until this spiritual home is found. Yet so long as the miasm is not brought to fruition, is not healed, it will continue to urge the person on toward endlessly new horizons. Home is symbolic of unconditional love and connection (*Mind; love; romantic, desire for*). Home is nearly the equivalent of love, as the place or the state of unconditional acceptance. It is where one can be oneself. On earth however the tubercular person, sooner or later, ceases to believe in the absolute love of themselves by others, or perhaps feels that human love is not sufficient, and they often divorce and remarry (*Mind; delusions, imaginations; loved, is not*).

Tubercular people are, like a tuberculosis patient, extremely sensitive both physically and emotionally (*Mind; sensitive, oversensitive; mentally and physically*). They tend to be interested in the arts and in them find an outlet for expression (*Mind; artistic; aptitude*). Most of the actors of the world are, by far, tubercular. Playing different roles on the stage is another way of constantly seeking change: to the point of changing one's identity and taking on another. The tubercular person has a longing to *find*, and therefore reaches deep into the souls of others, seeking genuine contact and mutual understanding. The tubercular process is strikingly analogous to the disease itself: like the mycobacterium in the lung which is encased into a calcified caseous tuberculoma, tubercular people tend to be too open at first, taking people into the depths of their spirit, only to be traumatized; they then "encapsulate" such experiences and carry them around for a lifetime.

The longilinear stature of anthropoid people expresses a tubercular reaching toward the sky, an urging toward heaven, toward the air element (*Generalities; tall*). The lungs connect our physical body with air. Air represents the spirit that moves in us. Through the lungs we inspire, receive our inspiration, and give back our love as *homo adorans*[46]: *Let every-thing that has breath praise the Lord* (Psalms 150:6). Air represents the spiritual, the non-visible, the nonmaterial—that realm which is higher than us, the realm of the sovereign God, *in whom we live and move and have our being* (Acts 17:28). The act of breathing is the act of taking in divine inspiration and giving it out. Second-circle energy, the circle of communication, presence, and love, is not possible when the breathing faculty is inhibited. The anthropoid morphology, with its tubercular base, predisposes to an innate second-circle tendency.

The *adumu* dance is part of the coming-of-age process for young Maasai men and it reflects such a heavenly striving. The Maasai people use the jumping dance as a showcase that signifies the strength of a warrior in the community. There are no drums accompanying the vertical jumps, but the men do chant as they jump. This dance is very important for the community—to be reassured that there are warriors who will protect the people as well as the livestock from the attacks by wild animals. The strongest warrior—the one who jumps the highest—is crowned and presented with a young woman who is ready for marriage.[47] He who jumps the highest is considered the strongest warrior.

The anthropoid, tubercular Maasai are a pastoral nomadic people subsisting almost solely on milk, meat, and occasionally blood. With the homeopathic understanding of tubercular preferences, it is not surprising at all—but instead confirming—that these are the chosen foods of the Maasai (*Generalities; food and drinks; milk, milk products; desires; Generalities; food and drinks; meat; desires*). As anthropologists have noted, in a natural environment abundant in a variety of foods which lends itself to successful agriculture, the Maasai choose to shun plant food and game meat. "How do we account," asks one anthropologist, "for the cultural

---

46   the worshiping human.
47   Evans Ntshengedzeni Netshivhambe, The crafting of Malende rhythmic motifs in indigenous Venda music with specific reference to Tshigombela and Tshikona dance – A fieldwork-based composition research enquiry. Thesis presented for the degree of Doctor of Philosophy in Music at the University of the Witwatersrand, 2019, p. 49.

choice to live exclusively on pastoral foods in an environment that so clearly offers alternative sources of subsistence?" This type of question addresses the dialectics of culture and practical reason, or the apparent "disconnect" between symbolic cultural traditions and materially efficient choices that seemingly promote survival. People's choices about how to construct their lives are usually not "rational," not consciously made for the sake of maximum economy and ecology. The culture of food and drink is not accidental but sacramental, in the daily ingestion and sustenance of the incarnated soul.[48]

People are, indeed, what they eat. Food choices derive from dominant collective cultural miasms or from dominant individual constitutional types (if a person is not part of a homogeneous culture, as is the case in many industrialized countries). Food is symbolic of an individual's or a culture's relationship with the earth/cosmos as nurturer and sustainer[49]. The significance of particular foods for a particular people is as inherent as language. As American Orthodox Christian priest and theologian Alexander Schmemann wrote:

> Centuries of secularism have failed to transform eating into something strictly utilitarian. Food is still treated with reverence.... To eat is still something more than to maintain bodily functions. People may not understand what that "something more" is, but they nonetheless desire to celebrate it. They are still hungry and thirsty for sacramental life.[50]

---

48   For an in-depth analysis of the ideational dimension and symbolic construction of the Maasai diet, see: Århem, K. (1989). "Maasai Food Symbolism: The Cultural Connotations of Milk, Meat, and Blood in the Pastoral Maasai Diet." *Anthropos*, 84(1/3), 1-23.
49   A circumspect analysis of the meaning of food in people's lives: Fox, Robin (2014). "Food and Eating: An Anthropological Perspective." *Social Issues Research Center.*
50   Alexander Schmemann. *For the Life of the World.* (St. Vladimir's Seminary Press, 1973).

Food—and not only any food but specific foods—imparts meaning into the daily rituals of eating and drinking. For Orthodox Christians, that for which we hunger and thirst is God's love and the recovery of our divine image in which we were made, making our most important food the Eucharist—Christ's body. For Christians, people are created in God's image and therefore maintain divine qualities, albeit hidden under the veil of sin. The taking of Christ's body in the Eucharist therefore becomes the ultimate homeopathic medicine: and via the law of similars this medicine intensifies or multiplies (however temporarily) these qualities. This belief is found not only among Christians. Anthropologists have long observed that many pre-industrial peoples believe that by ingesting certain foods, the person eating acquires the characteristics of that food. Homeopathically, we know that a person can't acquire traits that were never there; the characteristics of a chosen food instead resonate with similar characteristics in the eater, thus intensifying them. This is homeopathy.

The Maasai diet reflects perfectly the tendencies of the tubercular miasm and the anthropoid morphology. The Maasai consume mostly milk, meat, and blood. Meat is consumed only as a ritual food on special occasions. Milk, however, is the staple of the Maasai diet and often replaces solid food. The Maasai have been observed to maintain the physiologic ability for milk consumption by their genetic persistence of lactase, the enzyme necessary for lactose (milk) digestion[51]. This enzyme disappears in most people of the world at around age five, rendering milk in its pure form not wholly digestible. Milk has long been part of the traditional treatment of tuberculosis. Many cultures of the industrialized world still give warm milk for the treatment of lung diseases. Milk in the lactating mother is made by her blood. The Maasai drink the blood of their cattle on certain occasions; it is consumed by warriors to regain strength, and is taken from the cattle in amounts not large enough to harm the animal. Blood has a special place in the tubercular miasm

---

51   Nowak, J.K.; Dybska, E.; Dworacka, M.; Tsikhan, N.; Kononets, V.; Bermagambetova, S.; Walkowiak, J. Ileal "Lactase expression associates with lactase persistence genotypes." *Nutrients* 2021, 13, 1340.

as symbolic of the life force, of the most vital part of the person, associated with the soul's life as given by God. Children for whom this miasm is dominant desire milk and meat more than any other miasm. They also desire fat. Blood has a significant place in the tubercular miasm also in that people for whom this miasm is dominant tend to bleed excessively: nosebleeds, bleeding wounds, uterine hemorrhages.

All of these miasmatic tendencies can be deduced through examination of the morphology.

Joint hypermobility

Second to the android morphology, people of anthropoid and anthropoid-gynecoid mix tend to have hypermobility of joints and ligament laxity. Whereas for the android type this laxity is most evident in the hyperextended knees, for the anthropoid group it is especially noticeable in the first three criteria of the Beighton score: passive apposition of the thumbs to touch the flexor aspect of the forearm; passive dorsiflexion of the 5th fingers beyond 90°; and hyperextension of the elbows beyond 10°. In addition, these people can easily touch the floor with flat palms and knees straight, without feeling discomfort. These traits are most often noticed in children, who also tend to be lean (despite having good appetites) and emotionally excitable, often tending toward hyperactivity. Such children have an inborn ability for ballet and gymnastics, although many specialists don't recommend these activities for people with hypermobile joints, positing that such exercises can make the problem worse.

Mineral and micronutrient assimilation: excess or deficit?

The anthropoid and anthropoid-gynecoid mix types tend to have problems assimilating micronutrients from conception. Their lean build and spare bones speak of this. In infants, teeth come in later than average, sometimes as late as one year of age. They learn to walk independently often only after 12–14 months. They are prone to rickets or, if not outright rickets, symptoms that often accompany rickets: atopic dermatitis, excessive perspiration, late closure of fontanel, flaccid muscle tone, anemia. These symptoms are not for lack of intake. Homeopathic understanding offers monumental rethinking about traditional cause-and-effect concepts, and this rethinking is most relevant for the field of nutrition. The classic example is the subject of rickets. Rickets is believed to be caused by vitamin D deficiency, leading to inefficient assimilation of calcium and phosphorus and improper bone mineralization. There are however many paradoxical statistics: for example, rickets is more common in areas of the world where sunlight is abundant. Traditional medicine attributes this to a higher level of melanin in the skin, preventing adequate absorption of ultraviolet rays; or to the practice of using excessive bodily coverings (really only applicable to Muslim women in areas where full body covering is the norm). In more northern climes, the lack of sunlight is attributed to staying indoors too much or using too much sunscreen! Among North American children, rickets is more common in breastfed babies of non-White mothers. The standard explanation would likely attribute this to the degree of melanin in the skin and reduced sun exposure. We however argue for the constitutional approach. What is the homeopathic-morphological approach to such a phenomenon?

Homeopathy teaches to think in images and totalities, using symbols as tools to understanding the whole picture. Vitamin D supplementation is recommended across the board to nursing mothers and to their infants. This practice continues, despite the lack of evidence for it having an effect on prevention of rickets:

> For breastfed infants, vitamin D supplementation 400 IU/day for up to six months increases 25-OH vitamin D levels and reduces vitamin D insufficiency, but there was insufficient evidence to assess its effect on vitamin D deficiency and bone health. For higher-risk infants who are breastfeeding, maternal vitamin D supplementation reduces vitamin D insufficiency and vitamin D deficiency, but there was insufficient evidence to determine an effect on bone health. In populations at higher risk of vitamin D deficiency,

vitamin D supplementation of infants led to greater increases in infant 25-OH vitamin D levels, reductions in vitamin D insufficiency and vitamin D deficiency compared to supplementation of lactating mothers. However, the evidence is very uncertain for markers of bone health. Maternal higher dose supplementation ($\geq$ 4000 IU/day) produced similar infant 25-OH vitamin D levels as infant supplementation of 400 IU/day. The certainty of evidence was graded as low to very low for all outcomes.[52]

Instead of supplementing with vitamin D with the hope of improving absorption of trace minerals, the homeopath prescribes the constitutional remedy that covers the symptom-totality of the infant. Infants and small children reflect the mineral realm of remedies more than any other age group, in correspondence with their stage of development. Their main task is the creation of structure, a solid and reliable physical foundation. Their souls are "grounding" themselves to life on earth in physical bodies and undergoing growth at incredible speed.

In homeopathy we know that deficit and overdose of mineral substances exhibit similar symptoms like two sides of the same coin. People who have symptoms of mineral deficiencies—just like people who "attract" certain illnesses to themselves—do so because it is their constitutional predisposition, their weakness. For such people, taking supplements of trace minerals is interpreted by the organism as an extremely high dose, since their constitution resonates with the overall mineral picture, and can potentially cause serious aggravation of symptoms. This same phenomenon explains why some people react severely to the BCG[53] vaccine: the "small" dose of tuberculinum is received by a person with a tubercular constitution as an enormous insult due to the energetic resonance that takes place, and as a result the person often develops tubercu-

52   Tan ML, Abrams SA, Osborn DA. (2020). "Vitamin D supplementation for term breastfed infants to prevent vitamin D deficiency and improve bone health." *Cochrane Database of Systematic Reviews*, Issue 12. Art. No.: CD013046. DOI: 10.1002/14651858.CD013046.pub2.
53   BCG, or bacille Calmette-Guerin, is a vaccine for tuberculosis (TB) disease. https://www.cdc.gov/tb/publications/factsheets/prevention/bcg.htm

losis-like symptoms—some of which leave their mark for years. This is a paradoxical situation, since the very people who seem to need a certain substance (or in the case of vaccination, the very people who are susceptible to developing tuberculosis) are most at risk of taking the substance in a "material" dose. A homeopathic (dynamized) dose, however, produces the needed effect, bringing about the mildest intensification of symptoms and thus bringing them to (at least a relative) fruition.

In childbirth

The shape of the anthropoid pelvis predisposes to an occiput-posterior position of the fetus. If the overall size of the pelvis is large enough, there are no barriers to natural birth, especially if the baby's father is also anthropoid, since the baby's head will have the characteristic anthropoid form. The inlet of the anthropoid pelvis is oval, and the anteroposterior diameter is much longer than the transverse diameter. The front of the pelvis is slightly narrower than the back.

The sacrum deviates backward and, although flat, the posterior sagittal dimensions are long in all pelvic planes. Therefore, the space for accommodating the fetal occiput is larger in the back of the pelvis than in the front. The anthropoid pelvis has the largest sacrum of all morphological types, often noted as having not the typical five, but six fused vertebrae, so it is the deepest. The sacrosciatic notch is of medium height, but very wide, allowing four finger breadths to measure the sacrosciatic ligament between the ischial spine and the sacrum. The walls of the pelvis are often slightly convergent. The ischial spines are usually pronounced, but not encroaching, and the transverse diameter of the cavity is smaller than that of the gynecoid type, but not as narrow as that of the android. The pubic arch is a bit narrow, but this is offset by the fact that the outlet is very large. However, such a "high" perineum is prone to tearing.

Although the baby remains occiput-posterior in most labors with anthropoid morphology, this should by no means be regarded as pathological. The *implicate intent* of this morphology, together with the person's dominant miasm and constitution, clearly have meaning and purpose built in. Our task is to identify what we are observing and to support the entire process for what it is. Labor for this morphological type is generally less complicated than for the android morphology, in which occiput-posterior babies are also common. The differences are many and are easily identifiable, as described in this table:

	Anthropoid	Android
General body build	Narrow and lean	Heavy-set
Leg shape and length	Straight from hip to foot	Convergent from hip to knee then divergent
Face and head shape	Dolicocephalic	Round head, sometimes brachycephalic
Shoe size	Large	Small
Bone mass	Fine	Massive
Pelvic depth	Quite deep	Average–deep
Pelvic shape from top to bottom	Mildly convergent	Quite convergent, funnel-shaped
Perineum length	Long	Long
Transverse diameter of the midpelvis	Average—reduced	Average—reduced
Carries the baby	Out front and low	Inside and high

Anthropoid morphology in voice and presence work

Among performers there is a high proportion of anthropoid morphological types. Their slender, graceful lines and longilinear features make them appealing choices in professions for which physical attraction is valued. They have a natural talent for ballet and dance, and for sports that require stamina, jumping, and plasticity of movement. In voice and presence work they display a high level of self-confidence and love for the discipline, and rarely are hindered much by being afraid of the audience. They are the thoroughbred racehorses of morphological types. While usually very second circle in their level of presence, they can sometimes seem to have such a fierce reaching for the sky that they lose grounded-ness, which can lead to "resting on their laurels." Gentle reminders of the need to keep working however are often all that is needed to inspire them to persist in their efforts. Like all tubercular types, they have stamina for the sprint run and then get tired. In birth too, an anthropoid woman will exhibit extravagant enthusiasm and delight until the end of the dilation phase, at which point she might fall into a deep sleep, the "calm before the storm." In voice work these individuals need to ensure they get adequate rest—otherwise burnout is inevitable.

Cases

Case 1: Donna

Donna came to see me for a natural birth after three cesarean sections. For each of her three previous pregnancies the doctor had allowed for a "trial of labor," but every birth ended operatively due to failure of the baby to descend. All three children were boys weighing over 4 kg (8.5 lbs), and all were occiput-posterior. She had, additionally, carried each baby to 42 weeks' gestation. Her labor had always been strong, with regular and effective contractions up until full dilation of the cervix, at which point none of the babies descended below the level of the midpelvis.

On morphological examination, Donna was found to have an anthropoid pelvis. We discussed all the options and concluded that her chances of giving birth vaginally would increase under the following conditions: 1) labor begins by her estimated due date, so that the baby's skull bones are more moldable; 2) giving birth by 40 weeks increased the probability that the baby will be smaller; 3) we would need to receive the blessing of my backing obstetrician in order to attempt a home birth. Donna readily agreed to this reasoning and having received the green light from my backup, she took 220 ml. of castor oil at 40 weeks with the intention of inducing contractions.

After a few hours, Donna found herself frequenting the toilet, and the contractions began after 2 hours. When I arrived at her home, she was having contractions every 10 minutes, and her cervix was dilated to 5 cm and completely effaced. The baby was in the LOA (left occipital anterior) position. She decided to lie down to rest, as it was the middle of the night. Within 30 minutes I heard moans and grunting coming from the bedroom and straining sounds. I hurried to check on her and upon examination was surprised to find full dilation and baby's head on the pelvic floor.

She nimbly got up, went into the inflatable pool, resolutely sat down in a squat, and before I could utter a word of caution to attempt to slow the process, she made a house-shattering "Oooooooaaaaahhhhh-hhhh!" and her baby exploded into the water. I succeeded in catching the baby girl as she burst into life, then placed her on her mother's chest. Donna herself was astounded, as were the other family members who came into the room wiping the sleep from their eyes to greet the new family member. Labor had lasted three hours from start to finish. In keeping with her morphology with its characteristic "high" perineum and owing to the speed of the delivery, Donna suffered a second-degree tear, which was easily sutured, and the postpartum period passed without problems.

Case 2: Katie

Katie was pregnant with her second child. She gave birth to her first baby in a birthing center, and labor had been induced at 40 weeks' gestation for suspicion of a "large baby." This prognosis notwithstanding, she had given birth to a healthy girl weighing 3700 grams (8 lbs 2 oz). Now she sought natural birth.

Katie had the kind of model figure that many women envy: she was slender and long limbed, graceful, elegant, and beautiful. All her childhood Katie had studied ballet and had been forced to give it up after an accident on stage that involved a torn ligament. In recent years, though, she had found great joy and self-actualization in motherhood. She remained active her entire pregnancy and indeed practiced yoga for many years, which continued during pregnancy.

Her labor began with spontaneous rupture of the membranes at 40 weeks and 2 days gestation and the baby in the right occiput-posterior position. Within a couple hours her contractions started and intensified quickly, and when I arrived at her house her cervix was already 7 cm dilated. Katie paced the floor in between contractions. She was turned inward, concentrating all her energies on breathing as the contractions were quite intense and long. Three hours after contractions had started, her cervix was fully dilated, and I could feel the large anterior fontanel at 2:00 in her cervix. The baby's head was still relatively high at "0" station. During a contraction it did not budge in the direction of the pelvic cavity. Katie did not feel the urge to push. I recommended that she lie on her right side for periods of 20 minutes or so and alternate this position with walking, being sure to have her visit the toilet every 20 minutes or so to keep her bladder empty.

An hour passed with no change in progress. On examination I found the baby's head to be in the very same position. I encouraged Katie to remain on her side, getting up only to urinate occasionally. Another hour went by. The contractions had become weaker after the first hour of second stage, and I knew that best policy would be to keep her relaxed, on her side, allowing the internal "spring" of her body to wind up tight, gaining strength, until it would once again make a comeback with powerful contractions. This became evident after about 2 hours and 20 minutes into second stage. Katie's uterus began rising up high in the fundus during contractions and clearly exerting downward and outward pressure at the peak of them. Katie was starting to grunt at the end of contractions. I encouraged her to continue breathing through them as much as possible, pushing only when she couldn't hold back any longer. This gentle approach to the descent of an occiput-posterior baby prevents hypoxia and undue pressure on the baby's head.

After a long three hours of second stage, the baby's head finally appeared at the outlet, and at this point Katie could hold back no longer and pushed her son into the world, lying on her side, in one long contraction. He was born face-to-pubes, direct occiput-posterior, weighing 4400 grams (9 lbs 7 oz).

CHAPTER NINE.

Platypelloid Morphology

Women with platypelloid pelves have historically been associated with a contracted pelvis and a history of rickets. For obstetricians of times gone by, this was the relevant issue when met with a pelvis that was excessively flat or short in the anteroposterior diameter. Diseases such as tuberculosis of the bones, poliomyelitis, spondylolysis, severe congenital dysplasia of the hip with lack of bone formation, and similar conditions usually leave their mark in this way. Lordosis or severe scoliosis may also be observed. Such women may have a pendulous abdomen, stand, lie down, or walk in a strange way, and be of very short stature. Such severe bone pathology reflects either the tubercular or the syphilitic miasm. The latter expresses itself as varying degrees of osteomalacia. Syphilis as an acute illness in a pregnant woman has this effect on her child, causing necrosis of bone. The most common expression of this phenomenon in congenital syphilis is the loss of nasal bones, creating a flat nose in the face which cannot be mistaken. Although we moderns are often under the impression that congenital syphilis is a disease of the past, since as an acute illness it is treated successfully with penicillin, homeopaths know that such miasmatic acute diseases might seemingly disappear to the eye and even to the microscopic analysis of the blood, but the miasm is carried down to the next generations. When we see a child or an adult with the characteristic flat nasal bridge and upturned nostrils, we immediately associate it with the syphilitic miasm. Therefore, as in the case of the sycotic or tubercular miasms—which don't require active gonorrhea or tuberculosis infections in the parents—a syphilis infection in the parental history is not "required" to diagnose the syphilitic miasm in a child. The homeopath will identify it via morphological and constitutional characteristics. All the better, since most people are not informed about their parents or grandparents having had a venereal disease in any case!

Truly platypelloid women, therefore, represented in the day of Caldwell and Moloy a tiny percentage of all pelvic types (3%) and in fact cannot be grouped with the other types, insofar as such a phenomenon expressed pathology and not simply normal variation. For our purposes

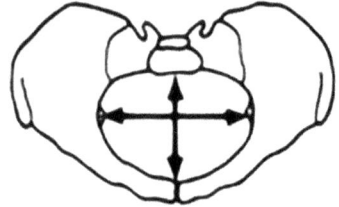

Normal platypelloid pelvis

however it is more relevant to identify a generally platypelloid tendency and grasp its expression as an overall platypelloid morphology. The great majority of women and men we observe with this tendency are actually mixed platypelloid-gynecoid, and so our discussion is in relation to the normal variation.

The brim of such a pelvis resembles a flat (from front to back) gynecoid pelvis. It is the opposite of the anthropoid pelvis, the brim having a short anteroposterior and a wide transverse diameter. The front of the pelvis is therefore very wide. The sacrum is quite capacious, but has a posterior tilt, so the sacrum is short and the pelvis itself is shallow. The sacrosciatic notch is wide and flat. The walls of the pelvis are slightly converging. The ischial spines may be more noticeable than those of a gynecoid woman, but, due to the flat shape of the pelvis, this does not affect the course of birth. The transverse diameter of the midpelvis is the widest of all types. The pubic arch is very wide and the perineum very short.

This type of pelvis in its classical variation is found most often in eastern peoples. While standing, these people have a lot of space between their legs from the hip down to the ankle; the legs are relatively straight and do not touch when standing with feet together. In women, the breasts are average size. From the back such a person has very wide, but not heavy hips and flat buttocks.

This morphological type speaks of everything that concerns physical balance. The wide stance seems to naturally lend itself to a profound centeredness. Such a morphology can be observed in masters of the martial arts and, indeed, it is no coincidence that the techniques and philosophy of the martial arts originated in the east, where such a morphology predominates. The sacrum is the natural center of balance and the legs are placed automatically at a relatively wide stance, allowing the martial artist to be in a continuous slightly forward posture, the weight being borne on the balls of the feet. Thus, for people of this morphological tendency, maintaining second-circle energy comes naturally. The pelvis is actually open and balanced in relation to the earth, allowing for a spectacular groundedness.

The platypelloid type tends to reflect either the psoric or the tubercular miasm and, often, the cancer miasm—especially when mixed with gynecoid morphology. Cancer in its various forms is grouped under the term *malignancy*, a word meaning evil, hostile, bad, malevolent, harmful. The cancer miasm should not be interpreted as being more pathological or frightening than any other dominant miasm. It is merely one *tropos* of several that are possible and each one has potential for extreme symptoms. Like all inherited miasms, the form and degree of symptom expression is not fixed. Knowing one's general tendencies and understanding the spectrum of possibilities, both positive and negative, is enlightening and the knowledge can be used for prevention, as well as development of one's innate gifts.

Examining the miasm from the characteristics of the acute states with which it is associated, we can gain insight into an overall picture. Cancer cells represent mutated cells, cells that have moved away from their original design and display the following characteristics:

1. They replicate as exact clones of one another (organization, identity, structure, order).
2. They lack cell death (apoptosis) and therefore continue dividing endlessly (continuity, death/life, immortality, the unknown).
3. Grouped together, the mutated cells form a tumor (identification with a group, rebellion, self-assertion, obstinance).

4. The cells eventually disrupt the functioning of the organism as a whole with the potential to cause the death of the organism (anarchy, revolution, destruction).

5. The malignant process can be initiated by environmental factors such as toxicity; exposure to radiation or other environmental extremes; trauma; and often reflects a hereditary tendency.

When studying either a person's symptoms or symptoms brought about by a substance, homeopaths look for what is called the tension of opposites. Symptoms are nothing more than extremes—intense expressions moving away from harmonious calm. A symptom is always a compensation for its opposite state. This is how the vital force expresses itself in its drive to achieve balance. What we are observing at any given moment is the person's internal pendulum of the vital force, if you will, expressing itself in this particular swing. When the pendulum has enough momentum or force, it reaches its zenith, or its endpoint, and then falls toward the opposite side. When we add the stimulus of the similar homeopathic remedy to this force, we intensify its swing, causing it to reach the zenith sooner, thus bringing the symptom picture to a temporal fruition after which the "pendulum" swings the other way, i.e., the symptoms subside. And so the symptoms we observe as a whole in a person represent the totality of their vital force's attempt to bring their being to a temporal fruition, with the anticipated swing in the opposite direction and—hopefully—healing.

Every totality can be seen as exhibiting one general theme within which a variety of sub-themes are expressed. Different homeopaths envision different central themes for any given miasm, remedy, and even patient. In the cancer miasm the theme of immortality—and all its sub-themes—prevail. The cell "rebels" by mutating and then never dying. Such an act seems to entail an egotistical will to assert one's uniqueness while ignoring the needs of the collective; indeed, it implies an ignorance of one's role and responsibility within the group. In the cancer miasm however this other-ness belies an extreme insecurity, a conviction about one's forsakenness, which drives the person to proving oneself, to being without a stain, in order to receive love. Cancer miasm children often grow up in a strict home atmosphere in which the parents demand perfection without showing unconditional love. For such a child every mistake or "flaw" becomes a tragedy; they are obsessed with order and cleanliness, excelling in school and sports and creative pursuits. Their compassion for others and especially animals is extreme, mirroring their own sense of rejection. Outwardly adults of this miasm are driven, hardworking, empathetic, and creatively gifted. They often enter the fields of healing, social work, art, dance, and education. The theme of immortality represents a thwarted intuitive drive toward *theosis*—restoring the divine image in oneself.

Using the characteristics of a cancerous process as the model, we observe the following tension of opposites (rubrics of the homeopathic nosode *Carcinosinum* are used as examples from the Complete Dynamics repertory):

Characteristic	Compensation (opposing tendency)
Conformism (clonal cell division); adhering to the rules (Mind; responsibility; strong, or too)	Creativity (Mind; sensitive, oversensitive; arts, drawing or literature, to); rebellion (Mind; domination by others, ailments from, agg.; Mind; domination by others, ailments from, agg.; father, by);
Obsession with order, structure, and organization (Mind; order, desire for; Mirilli's themes; organization; Mind; rest; cannot, when things are not in proper place)	Messy (Mirilli's themes; dirty); love for chaos (Generalities; weather; windy, stormy; amel.)
Individualistic perfectionism	Desire for love, acceptance, praise by being "too good"
Cruelty, disregard for the organism and life as a whole (Mind; cruelty, brutality, inhumanity)	Compassionate to the point of extremes (Mind; sympathetic, compassionate, too; suffering of others, to)

Physical general symptoms of the cancer miasm include: desire for animal fats (meat, butter, dairy), and chocolate; desire to dance or to exercise often to the point of fanaticism, and feeling better from exercise; feeling better from being close to nature; generally a "warm-blooded" person. Cancer is related to the sub-theme of *relationship*: the parts to the whole and vice versa. A person for whom this miasm dominates is concerned (and often obsessed) with finding her place in life, in the family, in relationships; people of the cancer miasm have a special relationship with the earth. They love nature, natural fabrics and organic foods. They are not interested in the latest fashions nor in showing off their material possessions.

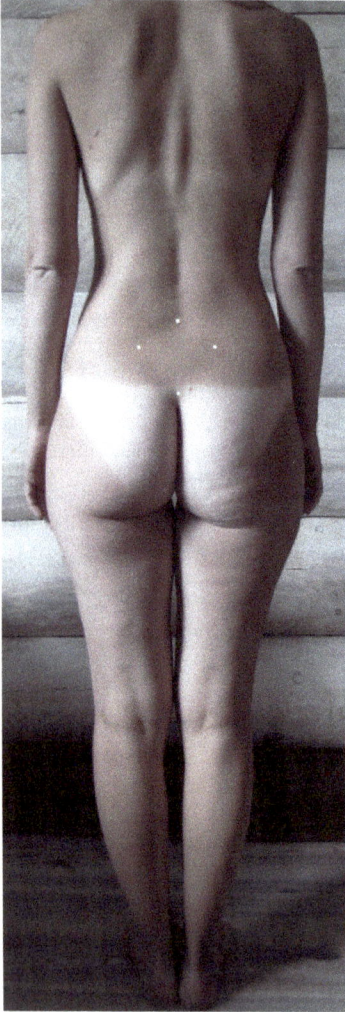

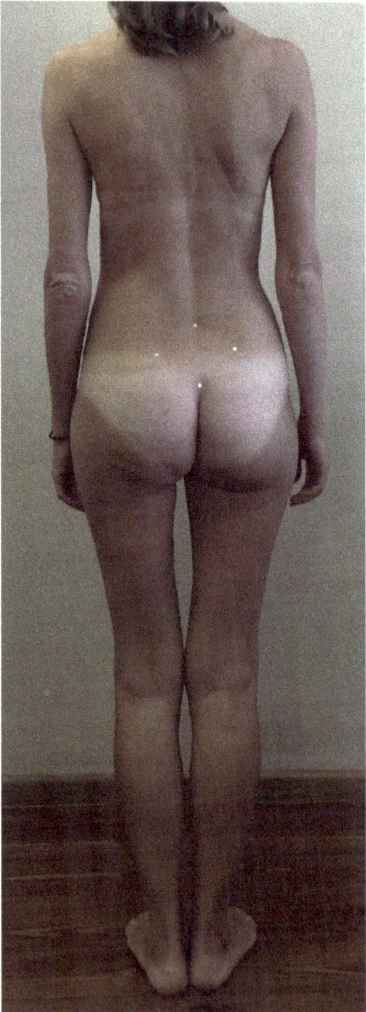

Platypelloid Morphology

In combination with the platypelloid morphology we observe a person who is driven mentally and physically and very close to the earth. They have creative abilities, are emotional, constantly interested in various subjects. They have a tendency to allergic reactions or simply sensitivity to chemicals or artificial food additives. In a compensated state, such a person is energetic, and in difficult periods tired, weak, and often sick. They are slightly sensitive to cold, although they need air and feel better at the seashore. There are many such people around the world now. The country of Belarus has an enormous number of people expressing the cancer miasm, possibly in connection with the Chernobyl accident of 1986 that left the country poisoned by radiation.

Many midwives and their homebirth clients are representatives of the cancer miasm. Women of the cancer miasm of platypelloid morphology make extraordinary mothers. They represent the typical "earth-mother." They are happy to give birth at home but only after thoroughly investigating all their options and studying the safety of it and interviewing the midwife in detail. During the period of breastfeeding of the first-born, these mothers are strong and cope well with household chores. They like to carry the baby in a sling, close to themselves, but this can adversely affect their backs. Due to the tendency to anemia, with each subsequent pregnancy they become more and more weak. Therefore, a diet rich in meat and dairy products is useful to them.

Possible problems in birth include disproportion and deep transverse arrest.

Cases

Case 1. Emma was a member of the Amish community near me when I lived in Iowa. She gave birth to her first child in the hospital without complications. Now she was expecting her second and turned to me for home birth. Due to the fact that Amish communities are relatively small and people marry only among themselves, some features of morphology have become characteristic. Emma's physical build was similar to that of many women in her community. On examination, I found her to have a large platypelloid pelvis and large bones. Her first child was born at 40 weeks with a weight of 3700 grams (8 lbs 2 oz). During pregnancy, Emma and I constantly adjusted her diet, which was distinguished by a large amount of cake, candy, and white bread. Owing to the fact that she found it impossible to completely cut them out, she suffered from chronic yeast infections.

When Emma started laboring at 40 weeks and 3 days, my assistant and I were glad because the height of the uterine fundus was already 40 cm and the abdomen circumference was 106 cm (the average girth measurement at 40 weeks is 100 cm or less; a larger girth suggests macrocosmic baby, twins, or polyhydramnios)[54]. An internal examination revealed 5 cm dilatation, but the head was directly above the pelvic brim and the sagittal suture was in the transverse diameter of the pelvis. It was so high that I could barely reach it with my fingers. In front of the head the bag of waters was bulging very low into the pelvis while the presenting part was barely fixed at the inlet. This state of affairs immediately concerned me because of the potential danger of cord prolapse. We waited, watched, and prayed for a normal outcome. Discrepancy between the size of the head and the mother's pelvis in a multiparous woman is a rarity, and I put all my hopes on this fact.

Contractions proceeded actively, strongly, and after a couple of hours the cervix was 8 cm dilated. However, the head still remained above the brim and the bag of waters pressed more and more down into the false pelvis. The cervix was hanging loosely around the head, like a sleeve, since the head was still not exerting pressure on it. I was now very concerned not only about the possibility of an umbilical cord prolapse but also about uterine rupture in the case of obstructed labor. The sun had already lit up the horizon of the corn field. A rooster proclaimed the

---

54   One valuable skill from classical midwifery allows the midwife to estimate the baby's weight by multiplying the fundal height by the girth (at the widest point) in centimeters, giving the approximate weight of the baby in grams. It is most accurate after 34 weeks.

Platypelloid Morphology

morning, and Emma's husband went to milk the cows. I went into the field, where a lone telephone hung on a pole 100 meters from the house, and dialed the number of my old Russian obstetrician colleague and dear friend, Anatoly. He was an obstetrician of the "old school" of classical Russian midwifery and always reassured with his calm, low voice. He recommended that I very carefully rupture the membranes, since the possibility of the head descending could be determined only after that. Returning to the house, I thought: wouldn't it be glorious if Emma could give birth herself on such a beautiful morning?

I explained to Emma the need for an amniotomy in order to allow the baby to descend. I gently explained that with such a procedure there is a risk of the umbilical cord prolapsing, and therefore it is necessary to do this while lying flat on her back so that I can determine the position of the head as accurately as possible and control the rate of water discharge. I also explained that amniotomy should be her decision, but that in these circumstances it is important to place a time limit, as the risk of rupture of the uterus will increase, and in the hospital they will immediately do the same thing. Emma said, "Do as you see fit." And having located the cervix, holding the amniotomy instrument in my other hand, I waited anxiously for several seconds. We were among endless corn fields, half an hour drive to the nearest hospital. All possible scenarios played through my head. Then, at the beginning of the next contraction, I ruptured the membranes. A huge amount of fluid came out right away, creating a deep puddle on the bed. Fortunately, by the end of the contraction, the head pressed firmly against the cervix and immediately began to flex. I left my hand inside, checking around the head for the presence of an umbilical cord, while my assistant listened to the baby's heartbeat. "Everything is in good. We are waiting for the next contraction!" At the next contraction, Emma became uncomfortable, as the head descended into the curve of the sacrum in an instant and exerted strong pressure on her anus. "Emma, everything is fine, you'll give birth soon!" We helped her get up and take a more comfortable position. After two contractions, the baby's head was on the pelvic floor and after two more she was born—a healthy girl weighing 4600 g (10 lbs 14 oz).

Emma gave birth again after two years, and the third birth proceeded in the same way as the second, only this time I knew in advance what to expect.

Case 2: Rosemary was also a member of the Amish community. She turned to me about an upcoming birth. Morphologically she looked like Emma. She'd already had 16 pregnancies (apart from the present) and 11 births. She was 38 years old. She gave birth to all her children in the hospital, since almost all were born prematurely. The previous birth occurred at 24 weeks, and the baby died a few days later. Rosemary still grieved for this child. She constantly called her by name. Despite the large number of children, she talked about every one of them with tender love and was happy about every succeeding pregnancy. However, this time she was very afraid to give birth before her due date.

From her history it became clear that Rosemary had a tendency toward hyperestrogenemia—she always got pregnant easily, had a short menstrual cycle, had several miscarriages in the early stages, and labor usually occurred at 34–36 weeks. I prescribed her a constitutional homeopathic remedy and wild yam in herbal form as capsules, 2 capsules 3 times a day until the 24th week of pregnancy; in addition, she rubbed her abdomen with wild yam cream and took 5–10 drops per day of Lobelia tincture in a homeopathic dilution of 3x.

Rosemary safely passed the gestation date at which she had lost her previous child and began to calm down. We continued to observe her more often than usual throughout her pregnancy, and when the expected date of her birth passed, we were joyfully surprised: for the first time in her life, she reached—and then passed—her due date! Contractions began at 41 weeks and 5 days.

The birth proceeded quickly, as expected. When the baby's head began to put pressure on the pelvic floor and there was a desire to push, abundant waters suddenly gushed out, and with them thick meconium. On examination, the cervix was fully dilated. The head was at +2, and the sagittal suture was in the transverse diameter of the pelvis. The baby's heartbeat was normal. Soon she felt the urge to push again and after three contractions the head was born, emerging in the transverse diameter, without having undergone internal rotation. In Rosemary's case it was an example of a capacious platypelloid pelvis, ample enough for even a very large baby to be born but with a flat anteroposterior diameter. The boy was born healthy with a weight of 4200 grams (9 lbs 3 oz), for which Rosemary was unspeakably grateful.

Platypelloid Morphology

CHAPTER TEN

Morphology and Occiput-Posterior Birth

Occiput-posterior (OP) position of the fetus is one variation of the vertex positions. Studies demonstrate that persistent occiput posterior position (in which the baby remains occiput-posterior and does not rotate occiput-anterior) is associated with a higher incidence of complications of labor and delivery. One study showed that only 1 in 4 nulliparous women and just over one half of multiparous women whose babies are in persistent OP position achieve a spontaneous vaginal delivery[55]. In this regard, midwives have come up with various methods to encourage the baby to rotate into the anterior position toward the end of pregnancy or during labor. In this chapter, we will analyze the issues related to the occiput-posterior position in the context of morphology. The subject is important not only for midwives but for any practitioner who works with pregnant women.

In which women does the OP position arise?

Statistics show that occiput-posterior position is observed in early labor among primiparous women (with the posterior fontanel at either 4:00

---

55   Anne D. Walling, MD. "Persistent Fetal Occiput Posterior Position." *Am Fam Physician.* 2004;69(1):191-19.

or 8:00) as frequently as half the time[56]. Nearly all babies rotate into the anterior position after the head descends into the pelvic cavity (and these can then be considered anterior babies). About 20% remain posterior until the head descends to the pelvic floor. About 5% of these babies will remain posterior until birth. Interestingly, among the OP babies who remain posterior until the pelvic floor, 18% occupy the right occiput-posterior position (ROP), and only 2% occupy the left occiput-posterior position (LOP). Current thinking explains this uneven division as caused by the presence of the mother's sigmoid colon on the left and the fact that the uterine muscles have a right-turning rotation. The predominance of the left occiput-anterior position (LOA) is explained by the same logic.

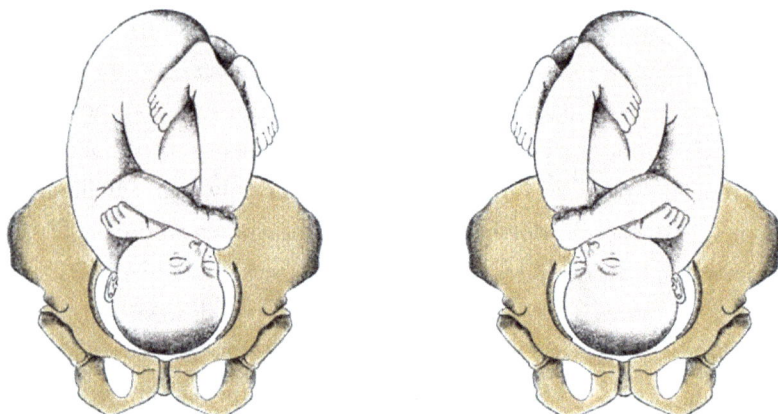

Fig. 1: Left occiput posterior (LOP) (left) and Right occiput posterior (ROP) positions (right)

Homebirth midwives in the era of modern medicine are characterized by some specific constitutional symptoms of their own: we enjoy a raw sense of life, a life without the current illusions of security. We have a burning passion to live—and that means experiencing life in its truest

---

56   Hulda Hjartardóttir, MD, et al. (2021). "When does fetal head rotation occur in spontaneous labor at term: results of an ultrasound-based longitudinal study in nulliparous women." *American Journal of Obstetrics and Gynecology*. Volume 224, Issue 5, May, pages 514.e1-514.e9.

Morphology and Occiput-Posterior Birth

form. Our passion for homebirth midwifery is fueled by this drive. Every woman in labor, every birth of a baby gives us a mirror in which we find our reflection and through which we experience a virtual catharsis. This catharsis serves us as an acute illness serves a chronic human miasm: to bring out our own symptoms and, in the end, to heal our lifelong "illness." We choose homebirth midwifery (or any other calling) not on the basis of conscious rational weighing of objective information, but subconsciously, on the basis of our inexplicable attraction to experience that intensifies our symptoms. This is the universal homeopathic process. It is a general observation of what people do. It does not have a "good" or "bad" rating. But when we realize what exactly is behind our motivations, desires, decisions, then we understand the objects of our aspirations in a different way. We begin to see our desires as symptoms, characteristics, traits that require maturation. We begin to see ourselves from the outside. We can then see other people from the outside, and realize that aspirations, choices, and behavior are not the person, but only characterize the person as attempts to an end.

From the perspective of a constitutional inclination toward an unsheltered life, midwives try to come up with and apply non-drug methods to resolve complex (and sometimes simple) obstetric situations. For the midwife, with a bird's eye view of our constitutional symptoms, a difficult situation presents us with a sweet challenge. These are calls to action. Our actions in solving a difficult situation satisfy the feeling of life and our direct participation in it. There is an irony in this: we midwives, at the beginning of our journey and with all arrogance, condemn those who practice the medical model of childbirth, sure that they "love to interfere," that they are "over-controlling" at every step. In fact, we home-birth midwives are, deep down in our constitution, just as controlling (if not more so); only the means of our control differ. No matter how much we declare that we are "sitting on our hands," we actively intervention at every turn. Many midwives refuse to care for women who are not ready, for example, to attend lengthy childbirth preparation classes. Others insist that her clients see an osteopath or chiropractor or some other practitioner regularly. Still others nearly demand that clients participate in meditation, yoga, or any variety of spiritual practice. Many midwives in Russia require their clients go to confession and communion at certain intervals throughout pregnancy and won't attend the birth without the blessing of a priest. They might insist on taking specific dietary supplements or bee products or herbs in a strict regimen; require specific exercises or psychotherapy; go to the sauna (another Russian practice) with a group of pregnant women regularly. They may insist that women give birth only in water, or only on land, and that an osteopath examine the newborn to correct the "birth trauma" of the baby. The list of potential recommendations of midwives is endless!

This is what we observe regularly in homeopathic practice. The human constitution as observed in any human being consists of extremes, each of which has its opposite side, and together they make up two sides of the same coin. Just how this information—these constitutional symptoms—relate to a discussion of occiput-posterior position will soon become clear.

In 1995, midwife Gene Sutton and childbirth educator Pauline Scott published a book in which they set out their theory called "optimal fetal positioning"[57]. This theory says that the modern sedentary lifestyle and the lack of physical work in women even around the house (for example, washing floors on all fours) predisposes a woman to carrying a baby in the occiput-posterior position. Adherents of such a theory suggest that the OP position is observed now more often than ever—and purely, they would argue, due to the depravity of modern women by civilization. They teach (and make strong but unsupported arguments) that OP position can be prevented. More recently, a similar popular trend has emerged, based on the Sutton theory, but with a claim that the new method is "broader." The inventors of the new method sell entire courses, books, and workshops on the prevention of OP position through physical exercises. Birth instructors, doulas, midwives, and anyone else can get "certified" in the "fetal rotation" exercise method. Unfortunately (and not surprisingly) the popular method is not backed by evidence.

---

57   Understanding and teaching optimal fetal positioning, Birth Concepts, 1995.

Statistics from old obstetric textbooks contradict the conclusions about the wrecked state of modern women and its resultant occiput-posterior position of the baby. A textbook of classical midwifery from the 19th century points to the experience of one then well-known midwife M. Oak: she noted that out of 1913 babies who were born in cephalic presentation, 558 were in the OP position during labor (29%). She worked in one of the early maternity hospitals in France in the 19th century, in which, as a rule, women of the lower socio-economic groups gave birth; such women led a very active lifestyle with hard physical labor[58]. Which begs the question: when did life become so corrupted by civilization that babies in the womb ended up in OP positions? It is well known that women with android morphology tend to carry babies in the occiput-posterior position, and anthropoid women even more so, with their reduced transverse diameter and elongated anteroposterior diameters in all planes of the pelvis. Is it possible to consider the Masai women of east Africa, all of whom have a classical anthropoid morphology, as "destroyed" by civilization? Would it really be correct to assume that the OP position in their case is somehow pathological?

Attempts to influence the position of the fetus during labor are not new. We cannot know, but we can assume that birth assistants at all times have tried to influence the course of difficult births by changing the position of the woman. Modern research, however, shows that the *all-fours or knee-elbow position and rocking of the pelvis do not promote the rotation of the baby from the back to the front, even when the exercises are started from 37 weeks*[59]. **Besides this, knowing that as many as half of all babies are at least "slightly" posterior when labor commences, and**

58   P. Cazeaux, *A Theoretical and Practical Treatise of Midwifery*, translated from the 5th French edition (Philadelphia, Lindsay and Blakiston, 1860).
59   —Kariminia, Azar & Chamberlain, Marie & Keogh, John & Shea, Agnes. (2004). "Randomised controlled trial of effect of hands and knees posturing on incidence of occiput posterior position at birth." *BMJ* (Clinical research ed.). 328. 490. 10.1136/bmj.37942.594456.44. —Levy AT, Weingarten S, Ali A, Quist-Nelson J, Berghella V. (2021). "Hands-and-knees posturing and fetal occiput anterior position: a systematic review and meta-analysis." *Am J Obstet Gynecol MFM*. 3(4):100346. doi: 10.1016/j.ajogmf.2021.100346. Epub 2021 Mar 9. PMID: 33705998.

knowing that most of them rotate into an anterior position sometime after engagement during labor, it becomes pertinent to ask: is there any sense at all in attempting to change a baby's position during pregnancy?

There are no accidents either in life or in obstetrics: there are only patterns. The explanation of any phenomenon lies much deeper than modern discrete, linear thinking wants to admit. A person does not come into the world as a blank slate to be filled, but is born as a unique inimitable soul with a body that incarnates one's essence. Homeopathic thinking offers a different perception of observed phenomena. Instead of causal explanations, we initially assume the existence of a life force— inherent in every person from God. We assume that there is a holistic ultimate goal to which every person moves, although not consciously. Every created being contains a latent intention, which is constantly revealed and fulfilled throughout life. As discussed previously, Aristotle coined the term *entelechy*, a life principle that guides the development and functioning of an organism. Entelechy is the underlying ultimate design or essential form that determines the personality and character of an individual organism. This is his or her "soul," non-material, formal, causal essence; it is internal and teleological. According to Aristotle, the soul or psyche is "a) the source of the origin of movement... b) end [*autes telos*]... [and] c) the essence [*auton tropon*] of the whole living body"[60]; in other words, the defining ontological essence of the organism[61].

The vital force is observed only indirectly through the expressed symptoms of a person. Everyone hides and then reveals a certain plan about the self, embedded in the person from creation. This *plan* is invested primarily in the structure of the physical body. The Russian biologist Ernst von Baer, arguably the most important telemechanic (and biologist, anthropologist) of the mid-19th century, used the embryological paradigm to characterize his point of view, arguing that there is a prior

---

60   De Anima II.415b, in McKeon 1941, 561. Peri Psyches 415b.

61   Josephine Donovan. (2018). "Between the Species: Subjects-of-a-Life, Entelechy, and Intrinsic Teleology." *University of Maine*, Volume 21, Issue 1.

information model that shapes the resulting unfolding of personality through the embryonic process. He called this the "forming force" and claimed that it exists in the egg before fertilization[62]. "This 'impulse' has a completely different character from its constituents.... The laws which it obeys are teleonomic rather than strictly mechanical." And he believed that "the *whole* ontologically precedes and determines its parts, the whole directs the organization of its parts."[63] Such statements confirm the homeopathic concept and definition of health of the founder of homeopathy, Hahnemann.

First we need to return to the basic concepts. What do we know objectively about the mechanism of labor? We know first of all that a baby is born by spiral rotation through the birth canal. The presenting part of the body rotates first, and is followed by all successive parts. We know that most babies are left occiput-anterior during pregnancy and labor. Therefore, the head of such babies rotates clockwise (when viewed from top to bottom from the brim of the maternal pelvis, that is, in the direction of exit). However, a small percentage of babies rotate counterclockwise: those who are in the right occiput-anterior (ROA) position. For the anterior positions, the situation is quite clear. And for the posterior positions? Among them, 90% are in the right occiput-posterior (ROP) position. Almost all babies in an occiput-posterior position make the "long-arc rotation" on the pelvic floor to become anterior and be born. The long-arc rotation sees ROP babies as rotating *counterclockwise* 135°; the LOP babies turn in a *clockwise* direction 135° to be born in the anterior position. However, of the LOP babies, most make the *short-arc* rotation, *counterclockwise*, and the sagittal suture moves into the anteroposterior (OP) diameter of the pelvic outlet, and, prohibiting any complications, the baby is born in the persistent-posterior position face-up.

The helical rotation of the baby through the pelvis at birth reflects a general trend not only in the anatomy of human beings, animals, plants,

---

62   Timothy Lenoir, *The strategy of life. Teleology and mechanics in nineteenth-century German biology*, 125.
63   ibid., pp. 125-128.

and many substances in the natural world, but also in the solar system and the universe itself. Almost any asymmetrical pressing or movement of any part of the body causes a rotation, and any rotation of any part of the body causes a helical or spiral movement. We can only move this way because most of the muscles in our body are organized in such a way that the fibers are aligned in diagonals that spiral around the joints, wrapping around the torso and limbs from top to bottom. This helical anatomy of the spine and torso is the source of our strength and agility, giving us the freedom to bend, twist, and turn, rotate around our central axis or around any point in space. It's what drives all of our movement patterns, from crawling to swimming, walking, running, and climbing. It is also what gives us stability, the ability to maintain a vertical central axis or resist any forces that might bend, twist, or turn us in some way that we do not want. When viewed in isolation, as they are usually thought of, they simply look like diagonal muscles. But when looked at sequentially, it is apparent that they wrap around the torso and spine in continuous spirals that cross the center line front and back; thick sheets and ropes of muscle and connective tissue weave a beautiful crisscrossed double helix[64].

Movement in space occurs in a predictable way and is associated with the spiral structure of our bodies. Is it possible to detect a certain orientation of a person's movement by looking at the hair whorls on the head?

One pilot study tested the relationship between facial hair whorl characteristics and behavioral responses in horses to a frightening stimulus. Nineteen saddle horses were classified based on whorl characteristics (height, lateral position, and rotation). Each horse was tested on a new object, during which an umbrella was suddenly opened. The turn response was recorded. Rotation of hair whorls showed a correlation with rotation response with $P = 0.04$. Clockwise whorls of hair were associated with a right turn, while counterclockwise whorls were associated with a left turn. There was no significant correlation between the

---

64   Simon Thakur, http://ancestralmovement.com/spiral-anatomy-and-movement-continued/

lateral location or whorl height of the hair and the direction of rotation (P > 0.05). In conclusion, the direction of facial whorls can be used as a non-invasive method to predict turning response in horses[65].

Scientists have studied the possible connection between hair whorls in the scalp and handedness. One study sought to address the question of whether handedness and scalp hair-whorl direction develop from a common genetic mechanism. They made the following conclusions:

> The general public, consisting of mostly right-handers (RH), shows counterclockwise whorl rotation infrequently in 8.4% of individuals. Interestingly, non-right-handers (NRH, i.e., left-handers and ambidextrous) display a random mixture of clockwise and counterclockwise swirling patterns. Confirming this finding, in another independent sample of individuals chosen because of their counterclockwise rotation, one-half of them are NRH. These findings of coupling in RH and uncoupling in NRH unequivocally establish that these traits develop from a common genetic mechanism. The findings of coupling between handedness and hair-whorl rotation in the general public and their decoupling in NRH clearly establish genetics as the cause of handedness, while the findings on the progeny of discordant twins favor a single-gene/locus model[66].

That is to say, scalp-whorl direction and handedness are "unequivocally" connected; however, the scientific literature to date offers no studies examining scalp-whorl direction and fetal position during labor and birth.

In the 1990s, during an internship program under my direction with American midwives in maternity hospitals in St. Petersburg, Russia, we conducted an informal study comparing the position of a baby during labor and the location of its hair whorl. We found that in almost all cases

---

65   Shivley, Chelsey & Grandin, Temple & Deesing, Mark. (2016). "Behavioral laterality and facial hair whorls in horses." *Journal of Equine Veterinary Science*. 44. 10.1016/j.jevs.2016.02.238.

66   Amar J. S. Klar. (2003). "Human handedness and scalp hair-whorl direction develop from a common genetic mechanism." *Gene Regulation and Chromosome Biology Laboratory*, National Cancer Institute, Frederick, Maryland.

of ROA (right occiput-anterior) positions during labor, the whorl of hair was located to the right of center of the occiput and more frequently displayed counterclockwise rotation (the same rotational direction of the baby as it spirals through the pelvis), while in the more common left-anterior position, the whorl was more often located in the center of the occiput and almost always had a clockwise rotation. Additionally, I noticed that babies with more than one scalp whorl (which almost always have opposing rotational directions) tended to change their position during labor.

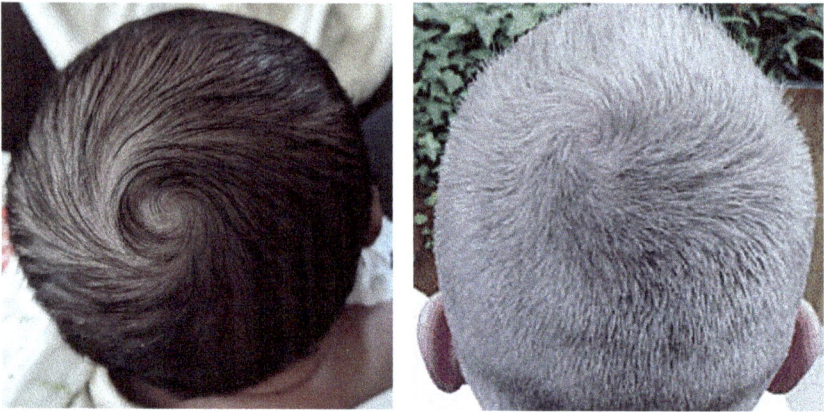

Hair whorls: clockwise (left) and counterclockwise (right).

It would be simplistic to think that babies occupy occiput-posterior positions during labor somehow accidentally or as the result of such minor factors as muscle tone and the mother's poor posture habits. Such an assumption already implies that posterior positioning is somehow pathological. It's time to delve into this very common obstetric topic and look at the question with new eyes. How we understand something determines how we will relate to it. How we understand a difficult situation determines how we deal with it. The position occupied by a baby in the uterus arises in connection with the individual characteristics of the morphology of the mother, in combination with the laterality of the child. My experience has borne out this conclusion. These factors are not random, but predetermined. They can most often be recognized from early pregnancy. The morphology of the mother can be determined in detail even before pregnancy. The laterality of the fetus is indicated with high degree of certainty by its position in the womb during pregnancy. The side toward which the occiput is facing (left or right) is usually noticed long before the onset of labor and is often persistent.

Other questions are also raised: how is the position of a breech baby related to hair whorls and laterality?

Labor

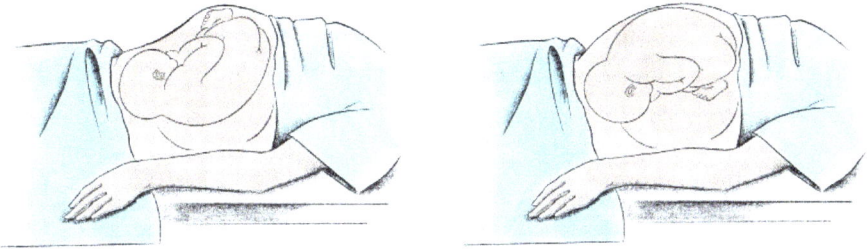

Dip in the belly (left) is characteristic in occiput-posterior position.

Recognizing the posterior position is not difficult: look for a saucer-shaped depression near the woman's navel. It is formed due to the "hollow" between the head and lower limbs of the fetus. The outline of the high, unengaged head of the baby outwardly resembles a full bladder (as seen in the illustration below). If the breech is easily palpable in the uterine fundus, the back in an OP position is difficult to palpate, since it is shifted to the mother's side, sometimes close to the mother's spine. The limbs are palpated on both sides of the axis of symmetry. At term, if the posterior position is more than slight, the baby's head is high; the sinciput rests on and above the pubic symphysis. This is due to the fact that a large presenting diameter, namely the occipital-frontal (11.5 cm) is rarely able to enter the pelvic brim before contractions begin, at which time relative flexion occurs. The back of the head and the upper anterior part of the head are at the same level. Only as a result of flexion does it become possible for the suboccipitofrontal diameter (10 cm) to engage in the pelvis, and flexion only occurs in response to strong contractions exerting massive force downward from above. Moreover, these babies are "forced" to turn into an anterior position only when the head descends to the pelvic floor; therefore, trying to force the baby to change from posterior to anterior at the end of pregnancy is pointless. The baby is literally directed through the pelvic planes during labor as it descends under the influence of contractions. The best way to handle occiput-posterior positions during labor is expectant management.

The 20th century was characterized by excessive medical intervention in childbirth. The current natural birth culture of the 21st century is often characterized by another form of unnecessarily complicating birth by asking the laboring woman to "jump through various hoops" in order to facilitate what is already in fact a normal labor. Perhaps this phenomenon arose as a defensive reaction against the medical approach to childbirth. However, the desire to improve the process should be prefaced by the desire to thoroughly understand the process, to the extent such is possible.

The OP position can cause problems mainly in the primiparous in which the cervix is not ripe by the estimated due date. In such a woman, the likelihood of premature rupture of membranes is increased due to uneven pressure of the head on the soft and hard structures of the birth canal. If, in addition, her baby is large, and she herself has massive bones and android morphology, the prognosis for birth is less favorable. She is likely to have a protracted first stage of labor and possibly secondary labor dystocia. Descent of the fetal head may slow down even with satisfactory contractions. A woman may experience a strong urge to push early in labor as the back of the baby's head presses against her rectum.

The descent of the head depends on the degree of its flexion; the diagnosis is facilitated by the presence of the anterior (large) fontanel in the anterior part of the pelvis, but in the presence of a *caput succedaneum*, it can be difficult to palpate. The anterior fontanel is determined by a four-sided diamond shape—the depression is easy to feel between the bones. The small fontanel has the shape of the letter "Y," but the recess is not palpable, since the bones are strongly compressed. The direction of the sagittal suture and the position of the posterior fontanelle help confirm the diagnosis.

Labor in OP position can be long and painful. The deflexed head of the baby is poorly applied to the cervix and therefore the negative feedback mechanism does not work as effectively to stimulate contractions. Contractions tend to become weaker and less frequent as labor progresses. A woman may experience acute, continuous back pain that is exhausting and demoralizing, especially when the progress of labor is slow. The ongoing support provided by the midwife helps the woman in labor and her partner to endure the birth. A midwife can provide physical as well as mental support, such as massage and other comfort measures, and suggest changes in posture and position. The knee-chest position, while not proven to facilitate rotation of the baby (insofar as it is forced to rotate only on the pelvic floor) can relieve a woman of some discomfort. Labor can be protracted, and the midwife must do everything in her power to prevent dehydration or ketosis in the mother.

A woman may experience a strong urge to push long before the cervix is fully dilated. This is caused by pressure from the occiput of the baby on the rectum. However, if the midwife encourages pushing at this point, it can cause cervical edema, which will delay the onset of the second stage of labor. The midwife can reduce the woman's premature urge to push by changing her position and demonstrating to her how to breathe. Most women during contractions ask for strong pressure on the sacrum, and intuitively take a pose on all fours. In such a case, *Kali carbonicum 30*, three pellets dissolved in water, a teaspoonful every 30 minutes, may be given until the woman in labor has taken 4 doses or until there is relief. Massage of the sacrum also helps. Immersion in water relieves the pain, but weakens the contractions, which is highly undesirable in an OP labor. Therefore, a shower is preferable.

Right occiput-posterior position mechanism (long-arc rotation)

- The position of the fetus in the uterus: longitudinal
- Head position: deflexed
- Presentation: vertex
- Position: right occipital
- Denominator: occiput
- Presenting part: middle or anterior zone of the left parietal bone
- The occipitofrontal diameter (11.5 cm) runs along the right oblique diameter of the pelvic edge. The occiput faces the right sacroiliac joint, and the upper anterior part of the head faces the left iliopectineal eminence.
- Flexion. There is descent occurring simultaneously with increased flexion. The occiput becomes the presenting part.
- Internal rotation of the head. The occiput first reaches the pelvic floor and rotates forward 3/8 of a turn along the right side of the pelvis, lying under the pubic joint. It is followed by the shoulders turning 2/8 of a turn from the left to the right oblique diameter.
- Head crowning. The occiput emerges from under the pubic symphysis and crowning of the head occurs.
- Expulsion of the head. The upper forehead, face and chin slide over the perineum, and the head is born via deflexion.
- Restitution. Following the birth of the head, the occiput rotates back again 1/8 turn to the right, as a result of which the head is again aligned with the shoulders.
- Internal rotation of the shoulders. The shoulders enter the pelvis along the right oblique diameter; the anterior shoulder first reaches the pelvic floor and turns forward 1/8 of a turn, coming under the pubis.
- External rotation of the head. At the same time, the occiput turns another 1/8 turn to the right in alignment with the shoulders.
- Lateral flexion. The anterior shoulder emerges under the pubic symphysis, and the back slides along the perineum; the body comes out through the movement of lateral flexion.

Variations for the course and outcome of labor:

Long-arc rotation and anterior birth: this is the most common outcome. Satisfactory uterine contractions cause flexion and descent of the fetal head, causing the occiput to rotate forward 3/8 of a turn, as described above.

Short-arc rotation (persistent posterior): The term "persistent posterior" indicates lack of anterior rotation of the occiput. Instead, it reaches the pelvic floor first and the upper anterior part of the fetal head turns forward. The back of the head enters the concave space of the sacrum. At birth, the baby is face-up.

Diagnosis of persistent posterior:

- In first stage of labor there are signs characteristic of any posterior view of the occiput, namely:
    - The head is extended, and the fetal heart is heard from the side or in the center of the mother's abdomen.
    - Descent is slow.
    - The cervix dilates slowly in the transitional phase (between 7 and 10 cm) and the "anterior lip" of the cervix is persistent (the part that is not dilated from the anterior side behind the pubic bone).
    - Contractions gradually weaken.
    - The baby moves a lot throughout the first stage of labor.
- In the second stage of labor slow progress is typical. On vaginal examination, the anterior fontanel is palpable behind the pubic symphysis, but this may be masked by a large caput.
    - A large occipitofrontal diameter causes significant dilatation of the anus as well as vaginal gaping, while the fetal head is barely visible, and a large biparietal diameter stretches the perineum and can cause excessive protrusion. As the head moves forward, the anterior fontanel can be palpated directly behind the pubis. The baby is born face-to-pubes. There is a

characteristic upward displacement of the skull bones with the location of the caput on the anterior part of the parietal bone.

- During the birth the upper anterior part of the head emerges first from under the pubic symphysis to the glabella, and the midwife helps to maintain flexion by preventing the anterior part of the head from extending beyond the glabella and thereby allowing the occiput to slide over the perineum and out. Then she straightens the head of the fetus, holding it with her hand and bringing the face of the fetus down from under the pubis. Because of the large presenting diameters, perineal trauma is common, and the midwife should look for signs of rupture in the center of the perineum. An episiotomy may be required in some cases to avoid a third-degree tear. If the signs were not detected early, the midwife may first realize that the occiput is in the posterior position when she sees the baby's hairless forehead protruding from under the pubic arch.

Possible complications in posterior labor

Complications are more common than in anterior births. They are as follows:

- Protracted first and second stages of labor due to the weakness of contractions, increased likelihood of transfer to a hospital for stimulation.
- Fatigue of the mother and fetus (and increased likelihood of epidural anesthesia in the hospital).
- Increased risk of fetal hypoxia and meconium excretion due to increased pressure on the head.
- Bleeding postpartum, as a result of distension, atony of the uterus and prolonged labor.
- Lacerations of the perineum and cervix.
- Overdistension of the pelvic floor muscles and possible injury (cystocele, rectocele) due to a long second stage and prolonged active pushing.
- Injury to the baby's head (cephalohematoma).

- In a primiparous woman with a posterior baby, pregnancy is often prolonged, in which case potential complications of postdates labor are added.

- Increased likelihood of surgery (forceps, vacuum extractor, or cesarean section).

- Deep transverse arrest occurs when the baby's head begins its internal rotation from the posterior toward the anterior but gets stuck in the transverse diameter of the midpelvis. Usually deep transverse arrest occurs after full dilatation, or sometimes at 9 cm. The stoppage of progress is detected when the baby's head fails to descend, the contractions weaken, and dilation of the cervix ceases. Deep transverse arrest can occur when the size of the fetal head is slightly large for the size of the transverse diameter of the pelvis (this can also occur in a woman with a normal pelvis size but with a large baby).

Physiologic occiput-posterior labor

The first stage of labor in the posterior position often proceeds at a normal pace until transition—about 7–8 cm of dilatation. Then contractions become less frequent and weaker. With good uterine activity by the end of first stage the hormones oxytocin and relaxin are released, which act on the woman in labor in such a way as to simultaneously intensify contractions and relax her. Signs of hormonal action are expressed in the fact that the stronger the contractions, the more the woman relaxes after each one, to the point of falling asleep in between. At the same time, the baby in utero also falls asleep, as indicated by the absence of its movements and periods of cyclicity (low level of heart rate variability). In this respect, the baby is protected from the stress of the last stage of birth, and in the optimal course of events, is born in sleep. Normal natural childbirth testifies to this again and again. The child is born, as if nothing unusual has occurred, slowly opens his eyes from a deep sleep, looks at his parents with a surprised yet familiar expression, and, finding his mother's nipple, soon falls asleep again.

It follows from this that with a weak release of hormones by the end of first stage, contractions do not become stronger but weaker; the woman in labor, instead of sinking and dozing between contractions, becomes increasingly restless; and the baby moves more and more. The baby's activity at this stage of labor is a sign of labor dystocia (i.e., weak contractions).

Full cervical dilatation in posterior position is achieved slowly. The midwife feels the "lip" of the cervix in the anterior region of the pelvis, behind the pubis: the thin edge of the cervix remains and the head fails to descend, despite its proximity to the pelvic outlet. The pressure of the presenting part on the cervix is uneven, and this fact contributes to the persistence of such an "anterior lip", but uneven pressure is not its main cause, and manual removal of the lip is therefore not the preferred treatment. The foremost cause of the persistent anterior lip is weak contractions. The painful massaging of an anterior cervical lip during contractions should be resorted to only as a last measure, and only after the midwife has done everything possible to increase the strength of contractions.

Birth attendants often begin counting the start of second stage during this protracted, nearly-fully-dilated phase. This last centimeter of cervix still does not give the midwife the right to assume that full dilation has already been achieved; second stage begins only with complete absence of the cervix. In the posterior position a long second stage of labor is characteristic. Due to the fact that the head descends more slowly, the labor becomes prolonged in comparison with occiput-anterior labors, and both mother and baby get tired. The midwife should do everything to preserve the woman's strength.

Complete internal rotation of the head occurs only after it has descended onto the pelvic floor. Contractions press down on the child, pushing him forward. The head meets resistance from the bones and muscles of the pelvic floor, which dictate the repositioning of the head. To facilitate (but not force) the baby's internal rotation, the woman is advised to lie on the same side as the child's back, with the top leg strongly bent and resting on a cushion. The horizontal position puts the least pressure on the child and supports the likelihood that contractions will become stronger, the baby will descend, and then turn.

The midwife may check the dilatation from time to time, but the most fruitful tactic during the second stage in a posterior labor is patient waiting. Frequent internal exams won't hasten the labor. Primary in the midwife's mind is the condition of the baby: the head is being maneuvered through a tight space, creating more intense head compression. The baby's head must be afforded ample time to mold, so as to best adapt itself to the arduous passage and emerge, still in a state of sleep. The best outcome can be expected by leaving the woman lying on her side in a dark room, alone or with her chosen support person (by mutual agreement), periodically checking the fetal heartbeat from her side so as not to disturb her.

It is not advisable to perform an amniotomy because the bag of waters protects the head from undue compression. However, there are times when the uterine powers are so feeble and delay the process so much that intervention is necessary to artificially stimulate contractions. Emptying the bladder, sometimes by catheter if the woman herself is unable to urinate, is also sometimes justified so that the head directly presses on the cervix and causes contractions to increase.

It must be understood that "failure to progress", or labor dystocia, is almost always the result of *weak contractions* in a primiparous woman, whereas it is almost always the result of *obstruction* in a multiparous woman. Rotation, descent, and delivery are facilitated only by strong contractions in the primipara. The contractions are therefore the first factor that should be assessed before blaming failure to progress on anything else in first-time labors. The midwife should do everything to enhance contraction strength in alternation with periods of rest: helping the woman into side-lying and then vertical positions; providing refreshments (sweet black tea[67]); and attempting to keep the bladder empty.

---

67   Sugar, as is well known in homeopathy, is an oxytocic. The medicinal effects of caffeine (in coffee, chocolate, or tea, as the woman prefers) and sugar produce an initial reaction of stimulation, followed by a secondary reaction of relaxation. A person's susceptibility (i.e. degree of similarity to a substance) determines the point at which the secondary reaction will set in as well as its intensity.

If the second stage of labor in a primipara can normally last up to two hours in the anterior position, in the posterior position, it can last up to three hours, and in a multipara, up to two hours. The midwife must constantly seek a balance for the woman between rest and activity. What is absolutely contra-indicated in posterior labor is squatting during the second stage, or asking the laboring woman to sit on a birth ball or birthing stool. The period of descent after full dilatation cannot be rushed. A continuous vertical position presses the baby's head even more strongly downward and is like forcing a round peg through a square hole. By encouraging side-lying and breathing through contractions the homeopathic law of similars is initiated, in this case deliberately "weakening" contractions as much as possible. After a time the body responds to this "winding up of the spring" by producing strong contractions that lead to the descent and birth of the baby. Side-lying is the foremost "treatment" for difficult or lengthy posterior births.

The lower the head descends onto the pelvic floor, the more pressure is exerted on the baby's head, increasing the risk of hypoxia. Therefore, the closer to delivery, the more often it is necessary to listen to the fetal heartbeat. As already mentioned, the head turns at the very last moment; this is seen by the appearance of amniotic fluid suddenly trickling out, before or during a contraction. There are cases when the baby does not turn, and the caput continues growing. There are descriptions in various obstetric and midwifery sources of attempting to turn the head manually: an extremely dangerous and unjustified procedure in modern midwifery. R.H.J. Hamlin described manual rotation using the fingers, exerting inordinate force on the cranial bones, in order to rotate the head[68]. The procedure was later included in a popular midwifery book of the 1980s. This procedure, it must be recalled, was recommended by Hamlin in 1959, at a time when operative delivery was still avoided at all costs, and the use of synthetic oxytocin for augmenting contractions had only recently appeared. It is extremely dangerous for the baby and should never be employed. Forceps are still applied occa-

---

68   Hamlin, RHJ. *Clinical Diagnosis in Labour.* (Edinburgh and London: E&S Livingstone Ltd, 1959).

sionally for "prophylactically" rotating the head into the anterior, but the usefulness of the procedure has not been proven. One study found that "prophylactic manual rotation of fetuses in occiput posterior or occiput transverse position, confirmed using ultrasound examination, **did not increase the rate of spontaneous vaginal delivery compared with no manual rotation.** Manual rotation of the occiput posterior fetal head early during the second stage of labor was associated with a significant 12.8-minute decrease in the length of the second stage of labor with no changes in any other maternal or fetal outcomes"[69]. With that evidence in mind, it only behooves midwives to forget about trying to force the baby to turn and instead relearn the practice of patient waiting.

Our goal in any birth is a successful outcome on all levels, physical and mental. In protracted labor, the midwife should assess the situation as objectively as possible and, if necessary, decide on the transfer of the woman in labor to the hospital. In the case of a persistent posterior position with no or slow progress, the likelihood of hypoxia and non-reassuring fetal heart rate patterns increases. The midwife must anticipate the outcome as early as possible and have time to transfer the woman to the hospital in time before mother or baby have become dehydrated or physically exhausted, so that the hospital staff can adequately assess the situation and provide the necessary assistance.

Food for thought

Homeopathic perception of symptoms, and common sense, suggest that for every symptom that arises there is some meaning: not necessarily as a pathological sign that needs to be eliminated as soon as possible, but as the solution "chosen" by the vital force. The vital force moves and expresses itself as it can, at a specific time in a specific environment and within a specific framework. These conditions limit its "choices" in solving any

69   Burd J, Gomez J, Berghella V, Bellussi F, de Vries B, Phipps H, Blanc J, Broberg J, Caughey AB, Verhaeghe C, Quist-Nelson J. (2022). "Prophylactic rotation for malposition in the second stage of labor: a systematic review and meta-analysis of randomized controlled trials." *Am J Obstet Gynecol MFM;*4(2):100554.

problem. Its overall task is to maintain or achieve equilibrium, homeostasis, in a person. Whatever it is, the vital force always strives for this preservation in all circumstances. Morphological types that predispose to a potentially difficult posterior labor and birth can be discovered during pregnancy, which at the very least gives both midwife and her client hints about what to expect. Our task is to support the actions of the vital force. By respecting its inherent purpose, caregivers gain a deeper appreciation for an innate purposefulness of the entire spectrum of human experience, in suffering and in vigor.

CHAPTER ELEVEN.

Other Morphological Combinations

Most people fall into the category of mixed morphology. Due to the large number of seemingly contradictory mixed signs, these variants are sometimes difficult to classify. The first and last criterion for the most reliable birth forecast in women is always the rhombus. If the rhombus raises doubt, the next criterion is the Soloviev index, i.e., the thickness of the bones. Fine bones can "forgive" even a pelvis that is clearly borderline in size. In voice and presence work the rhombus points to the morphology which points to the center of balance which indicates the center of breath.

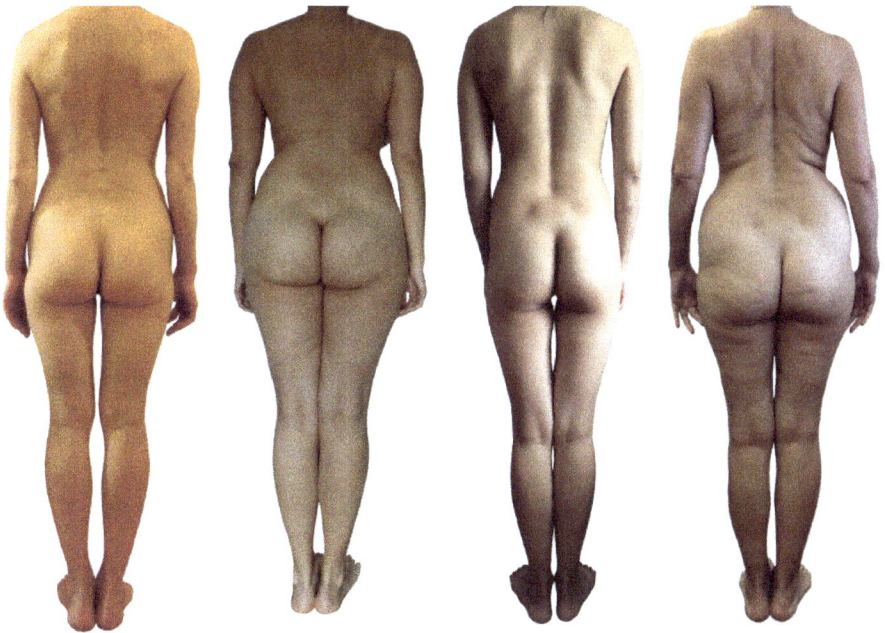

| 1 | 2 | 3 | 4 |

With mixed morphology, the rhombus is considered first and foremost, as well as the shape of the legs and the space between them and the length of the arms. We compare all the factors and draw a conclusion. The homeopath should be able to elucidate the leading miasm, which also gives hints as to the morphology, and vice versa.

1: A woman with obvious signs of gynecoid morphology: the waist is clearly defined, which the elbows clearly do not touch; legs are straight, converge and diverge in different places; shoulders gently sloping. But she also has some characteristics that are not typical for gynecoids: the shoulders are the same width as the hips; arms are longer than usual—lower than the lower edge of the buttock; between the legs there is not just a gap, but a real separation along the entire length of the legs. The rhombus is not clearly visible, but judging by the legs one can assume a very wide transverse diameter. As a result: mixed gynecoid-platypelloid morphology. This woman is of small height and weight, and she gave birth easily and quickly.

2: A nulliparous woman. She has a completely curvaceous shape: the buttocks are wider than the shoulders, the legs converge with a mild tendency to an x-shape; hands and feet are delicate. The rhombus, it would seem, is gynecoid, but small, as if it does not correspond to its general volume and growth. Her plumpness betrays her high estrogen levels, which may explain her gynecological problems and infertility. This morphology can be defined as "hypergynecoid."

3. This woman gave birth twice without problems. Her shoulders are wider than her hips; in general, her body is narrow in the transverse diameters, which indicates an anthropoid tendency. This trend is also visible in the shape of the legs, which extend straight from the hips and leave little space between the legs. The rhombus is almost square, and the anteroposterior diameter is slightly longer than the transverse one. This woman has a figure like a teenager, although she is in her 30s and has two children.

Other Morphological Combinations

4. This woman has a clearly visible rhombus and especially the points of the transverse diameter. Diamond shape, shoulders narrow in relation to the hips and slender legs indicate a gynecoid morphology. The nuance of this morphology is that the mass has accumulated around the hips, which indicates the width and overall capacity of the pelvis. This often occurs in menopausal women. If there are no factors indicating a different morphology, we can generally conclude that she has a gynecoid morphology.

Asymmetrical morphology

Every human body is asymmetrical. Asymmetry is a normal characteristic of every bodily system. Our asymmetry is related to our laterality not only in our handedness, but also in unilateral dominance of paired parts such as legs, eyes, brain, lungs, kidneys, breasts, reproductive organs, and so on. Symmetry implies the length of arms and legs; relatively straightness of the spine, presence of scoliosis or lordosis; the absence of additional folds in the waist area, under the buttocks, in the very gap between the buttocks and on the hips; symmetry of the shoulder blades and shoulders; the size of the feet.

Some people develop unilateral functional asymmetries that then influence overall body posture (usually not the other way around). Posture in any expression becomes the compensation by the vital force to restore balance. These postural patterns reflect the ease and difficulty with which people breathe, rotate, and rest with left and right hemispheric activity of the body. Like other morphological characteristics, posture is part of the overall totality of the person, the soul's strivings in explicate form at any given time.

Symptoms associated with severe asymmetry include: shoulder, knee, and back pain; migraine headaches; dizziness; confusion; chronic fatigue; tension of the head and neck; and even breathing difficulties. A person's habitual daily activities can accentuate functional asymmetry and pathological manifestations.

Earlier in this book we discussed constitutional/miasmatic patterns and how they are expressed in posture and manifested in a person's quality of presence. It is important to avoid making conclusions based on what we might expect, and instead, to strive to see what is before us.

When gathering photographs of women's shapes for this book, I made a surprising discovery: almost everyone with noticeable asymmetrical morphology gave birth by cesarean section. Such asymmetry is not always visible to the eye, but in photographs it is striking. I concluded that severe asymmetry—even in the presence of an otherwise normal morphology—is the strongest warning sign of potential problems in a first birth.

Women with severe asymmetry often experience body pains and especially back pain, and often seek osteopathic or chiropractic help during pregnancy, which might ease discomfort, but usually makes no difference in regard to the course of labor. It is not always possible to influence the pathology behind the asymmetry during pregnancy. The great majority of asymmetry is due to congenital reasons and not acquired through poor posture. Congenital asymmetry is visible in such signs as: asymmetrical wrinkles underneath the buttocks or behind the knees; noticeable difference in leg or arm length; scoliosis, lordosis, kyphosis; torticollis; congenital hip dysplasia; pronation or supination of the feet; valgus (knock-knee) or varus (bow-leg) knees; rachitic deformations of the pelvis and extremities; various misshapen thoracic cavities (sunken chest—*Pectus excavatum*; pigeon chest—*Pectus carinatum*); flat-footedness; etc.

Body asymmetry is classically associated with orthopedic pathology, from mild scoliosis to occult hip dysplasia. When a woman has complaints or the diagnosis has been known since childhood, the task of the midwife is made easier.

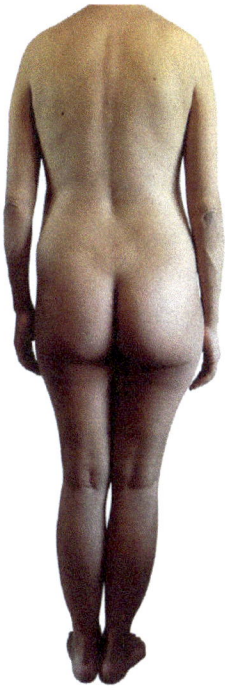
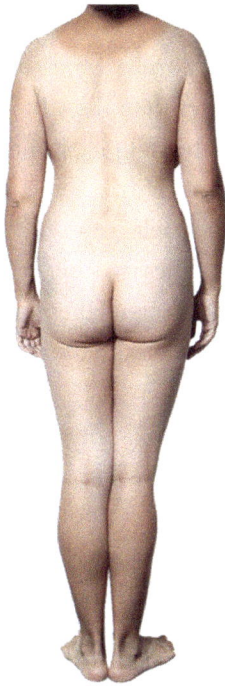
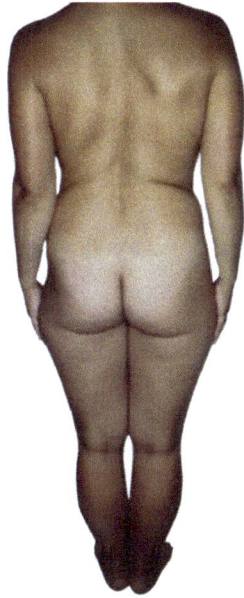

1

2

3

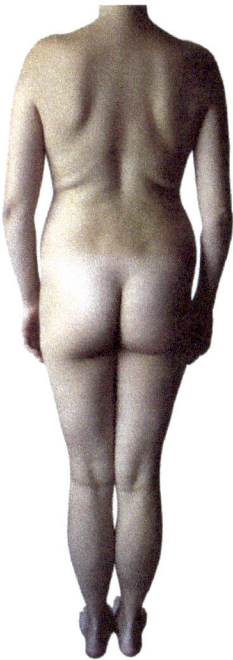
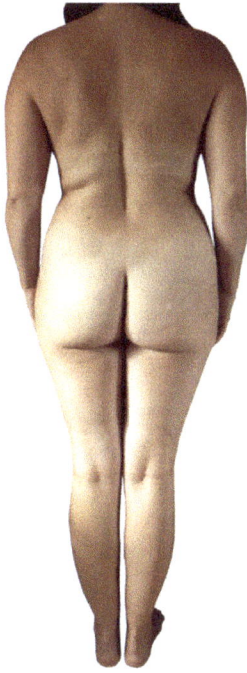
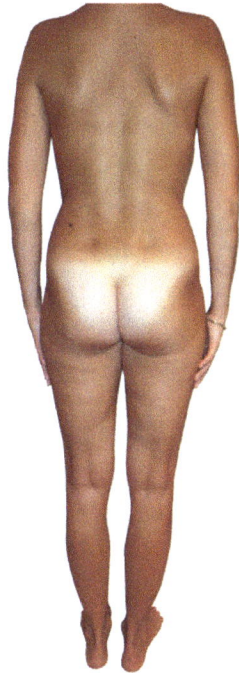

4

5

6

The birth stories of the women in the accompanying photos are as follows:

1. The right arm is much longer than the left; you can also see, by the way she stands unevenly, that the right leg is much longer than the left. This asymmetry undoubtedly affects the spine, which is slightly curved in the lumbar region. The pelvis itself is also curved, and this can be seen from the asymmetry of the hips: the right thigh is wider than the left. The rhombus is long in the AP diameter, and there is generally a tendency to mixed gynecoid-android morphology. In the photo she is in the last days of pregnancy before giving birth.

Her first birth began at 44 weeks of pregnancy. The woman was observed by a midwife and planned a home birth. The midwife assured her that going so far past her due date is not a problem and that she had nothing to fear. Her preliminary labor was excessively long, going on for more than 24 hours with no natural progression into the active phase and no cervical dilatation. At that point she had spontaneous rupture of membranes and thick meconium was revealed. It was decided to transfer her to the hospital. There they performed a cesarean section. The baby was born alive in a state of severe asphyxia and died a few hours later. Needless to say this experience was very traumatizing for the woman and her family.

The next two attempts to give birth naturally with a different midwife—despite the woman's newfound positive attitude after having analyzed her first labor and gaining a sense of peace about its misman-agement—also ended in cesareans, both times because the baby did not descend into the pelvis.

Morphology and Occiput-Posterior Birth

2. The most striking feature of this woman's morphology is the different leg lengths. Her left leg seems to be much longer than her right, and she can hardly stand with her heels together. The left leg seem s to bend under such an attempt. An additional fold of skin is observed under the left buttock. The gap between the buttocks is crooked. The arms are also different lengths. The rhombus is long in the AP diameter. The waist is wide. The gap of the buttocks is low. In general, asymmetric android morphology. Her first birth ended in a cesarean section.

3. This woman has clear asymmetry in the upper body. The right scapula sticks out and scoliosis is visible. The shoulders are broad, the buttocks are relatively small. The rhombus is long in the AP diameter. Morphology is asymmetrical android. The first birth ended with a cesarean section.

4. This woman's asymmetry is not as pronounced as the others in the photographs. Her rhombus is distinguished by the fact that it is extremely long in the AP dia ge, and her bones relatively thin.

Her first birth nevertheless ended in a cesarean section due to breech presentation. At the time of the operation, it was discovered that she had a bicornuate uterus, which was the likely explanation for the breech presentation. With her second pregnancy, she planned to give birth at home, despite the fact that the baby was again breech. She labored beautifully until full dilatation, even though the first time she did not labor at all; but at this point the midwife discovered a knee presentation, and since the baby was not descending easily, it was decided to call an ambulance and go to the hospital. There she gave birth naturally rather soon after her arrival. With her third pregnancy, the baby was in a cephalic presentation, and she gave birth at home with a midwife with great pleasure.

5. This woman has proportional gynecoid features. The photo does not show that the distance between the points of the rhombus in the transverse dimension is only 9 cm. Her height is 150 cm. She gave birth by cesarean section due to a contracted pelvis.

6. This woman has surprisingly pronounced points of the rhombus in the transverse diameter, despite the fact that she did not give birth naturally; she had a cesarean section due to cardiac pathology. Her rhombus reveals a tendency toward platypelloid morphology: a wide distance in the transverse diameter and space between the legs. In addition, the upper part of the rhombus in the AP diameter is very short.

Morphological asymmetry, if noticed early (preferably before or between pregnancies) can sometimes be corrected. Various methodologies now exist that address the specific problems of what has come to be called *postural kinematic movement dysfunction*. The Alexander Technique, which has been around for more than 100 years, is one. It emphasizes self-development, in which the person learns to change long-standing habits that cause unnecessary tension. Another method is offered by the Postural Restoration Institute[70], an organization working since 2000. Methods such as these emphasize becoming keenly present within one's own body in order to first recognize habitual patterns of movement and then the relationships between various parts of the body that are normally taken for granted. These presence-centered therapies are being developed more frequently as people become ever more disillusioned with one-sided approaches to healing. Such practitioners also benefit from an understanding of morphology as discussed in this book.

---

70   https://www.posturalrestoration.com/about

Afterword

> *Love responsibility. Say: It is my duty,*
> *and mine alone, to save the earth.*
> *If it is not saved, then I alone am to blame.*

—Nikos Kazantzakis

Diagnosis is the art of discerning (from διαγιγνώσκω—"to discern"). The observations in this book represent my lifelong striving to hone this art. This endeavor has been motivated by a desire to see the holographic *whole* of a person through the smaller parts of the human body. Behind this was the preeminent desire to see God in the human person. Diagnosis can only be the discerning of a totality, never that of just a part. This kind of discerning is exceedingly difficult. It takes years of continuous rethinking—*metanoia*—having changes of heart.

Many generations now have been nurtured on a cognition that favors the parts at the expense of the whole. This dis-integration of consciousness is the ultimate symptom of cultural breakdown. It is a symptom of lack of presence in a society. The capacity for seeing the whole of anything—be it person, experience, place, culture, geopolitical event, literary or artistic work, illness, or God—is an uncommon phenomenon in current human awareness, requiring creative thinking. This once inherent human function has all but been extracted like a purposeless (and sometimes irritating) wisdom tooth.

Finding the patterns that could lead to discerning and diagnosing has meant, for me, returning to the basic questions: "What is health?" And then "what is disease?" But a basic anthropology of healing is necessary before even venturing into the questions. Nothing can be taken for granted in understanding life. We each need to find out for ourselves, assimilate what we feel to be true, and question every assumption.

Quantum physics spelled out in tangible terms what the ancients knew unconsciously about relationship: upon entering into a relationship of any kind, we change the overall whole. The healer part-ici-pates—literally, "takes his or her part" in the therapeutic relationship, influencing and altering the dynamic; the outcome (although technically in life there is never a final outcome so long as we are alive) is thus shaped and shared by all participants, and it is always a whole larger (i.e., different, unique) than the sum of its parts.

This underlines the level of responsibility each human being has in any relationship. We are each responsible. We are responsible for taking our part. As practitioners our part is discerning, but discerning has a process. It begins by *seeing*. Our duty is to *see, identify, accept, and facilitate* the journey of those who come to us for help. We recognize and identify after seeing. Once we have identified what we see, and given it a name and a face and a voice, then we accept it—for what it is, without judgment, unconditionally. That's the essence of our work. Only following that can we begin to facilitate.

About the author

Molly Caliger began her higher education at Columbia College, Chicago, in theatre, and then transferred to the University of Iowa, where she earned her BA in cultural anthropology and Russian in 1983. In 1989 she became a licensed midwife in El Paso, Texas, and later a Certified Professional Midwife. She founded *The Russian Birth Project*—an internship for American midwives in Russian maternity hospitals—in 1992, and in that year emigrated to Russia. Approximately 100 interns participated in the project over the course of 14 years. Molly earned her DHom (doctor of homeopathy) credential from The School of Homeopathy (Devon, England) in 1997 and subsequently was licensed as a Homeopathic Practitioner in Nevada (1998). In 2006 she founded *Tropos School of Classical Homeopathy and Midwifery*, which functions to this day as the only program in Russia offering a comprehensive, 5-year homeopathic education. In addition, she received a diploma in Orthodox Christian Studies (Cambridge, England), in 2011. She has published articles in homeopathic and theological journals, and has written three midwifery textbooks in Russian. Molly became a Patsy Rodenburg Associate in 2022, giving her the qualifications to teach voice and presence according to the methodology of world-renowned voice coach Patsy Rodenburg. She brings a lifetime of experience in holistic healthcare to her work both in her homeopathy school and as a voice coach, working with people from all disciplines and backgrounds. Molly lives and works between three countries: Russia, Greece, and the USA.

She can be reached by e-mail at: vis.vitalis.course@gmail.com

Index

www.ingramcontent.com/pod-product-compliance
Lightning Source LLC
Chambersburg PA
CBHW060040030426
42334CB00019B/2415